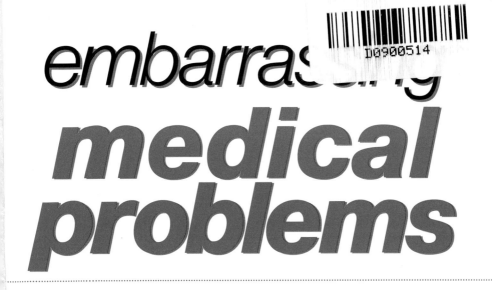

embarrassing medical problems

EVERYTHING YOU ALWAYS WANTED TO KNOW BUT WERE AFRAID TO ASK YOUR DOCTOR

Dr. Margaret Stearn

Foreword by Claire Rayner

Hatherleigh Press
New York

*embarrassing **medical problems***

Embarrassing Medical Problems

First U.S. Edition
© 2001 Hatherleigh Press
5-22 46th Avenue Suite 200 Long Island City, NY 11101
Tel: 800-528-2550
www.hatherleighpress.com

First published 1998 in the UK by Health Press Limited as
Embarrassing Problems © 2001 Health Press Limited

The publisher and the author have made every effort to ensure the accuracy
of this book, but cannot accept responsibility for any errors or omissions.

Library of Congress Information

ISBN 1-57826-067-1

Design by Andy Whitwood, Health Press Limited
Medical illustrations by Tek-Art, Croydon, UK
Printed in Canada

This book is not intended to be a replacement for proper medical advice and
treatment. In all cases, consult your physician.

Contents

Foreword

When I was a young nurse, I looked after a woman who died of embarrassment at the age of 43. She had been bleeding after intercourse for 3 years, and, she told the specialist, blushing all over, "I couldn't possibly talk to my doctor about such a thing, could I?" The only way she got into the hospital at all was by passing out in the street because she was so anemic. Oh, and by the way – that shameful bleeding was due to cancer. If she'd gone to a doctor sooner it could have been treated.

Of course the vast majority of embarrassing problems are not potentially lethal. No one yet has died of smelly feet or hairy breasts, or the possession of a banana-shaped penis. But a lot of people put themselves through untold misery because they "can't bring themselves to talk to the doctor about such a thing". It's more than a pity, it's silly – because no patient yet has managed to embarrass a doctor with a symptom (doctors are rendered unembarrassable by their education) so no patient need ever fear being embarrassed themselves. But no matter how often people are told this, still embarrassment lingers and keeps people away from reassurance.

Not everyone regards the same things as embarrassing, of course. One woman who will cheerfully discuss her smelly feet with her doctor may be so ashamed of having big breasts that she'll regard them as unmentionable. Which is tragic, because they can be glorious appendages to have. But it's the perception that matters: if you think something's embarrassing, then you might keep away from the good medical advice you need.

Hence this really splendid book. If you've ever let a portion of your own anatomy shame you, forget it. Just look up the facts in these pages and relax in the knowledge that it has to be a very common problem or else it wouldn't be here, so what can be embarrassing about it? You might as well be embarrassed about a runny nose. Oh, and if your problem isn't here, that's probably because you're the only person who thinks it's embarrassing at all. Everyone else takes it in stride.

So, read on and relax. This book is beyond doubt the most comforting you could possibly find.

Claire Rayner

Acknowledgements

It would not have been possible to write this book without the help of friends and Colleagues. I am particularly grateful to the following.

Mr Jeremy Wilson

Emeritus Consultant Surgeon, Queen Mary's Hospital, Sidcup, helped with the sections on the painful and itchy anus, and on fecal incontinence.

Dr Andrew Finlay

Consultant Dermatologist, Cardiff Royal Infirmary, provided advice on acne and on sweating.

Dr Rodney Dawber

Consultant Dermatologist, Churchill Hospital, Oxford, helped with the sections on baldness and dandruff.

Dr Graham Barnby

Dental Surgeon, Harrow Health Care Center and
Dr Philip Stemmer

The Fresh Breath Center,
helped with the sections on bad breath and teeth cleaning.

Professor Stephen Spiro

The Brompton Hospital, London, advised on snoring.

Dr Susanna Graham-Jones

Department of General Practice, University of Oxford, advised on how to talk to your doctor.

I would also like to thank the many patient support groups who read sections of the manuscript and provided invaluable advice from the sufferer's viewpoint. Particular thanks to the British Stammering Association for providing the information on page 150, which is taken from their leaflet *The Adult Who Stammers,* to Dr James Bingham for the illustration on page 100 and to Michael Dixon for general advice.

Author's preface

The aim of this book is simple – to help you deal with health problems that worry you and that are difficult for you to discuss with anyone. Almost none of the problems in this book are life-threatening in any way. Most are not painful. Yet they are not frivolous or trivial – they can profoundly affect your happiness and your perception of yourself. In the following pages I try to explain each problem, and tell you how you can deal with it yourself and what your doctor has to offer. See the ends of sections for lists of 'Useful contacts' who can provide further information and advice.

Why do we feel embarrassed about certain matters and not about others? Many of the things that embarrass us are completely natural, but modern society seems to have decreed they are unacceptable. Take 'wind' for example – we all produce more than a pint of intestinal gas a day, but most of us feel embarrassed if we fart noticeably. If we were still Stone Age hunter-gatherers spending most of our time outside we wouldn't worry about passing wind whenever we felt like it. The same goes for sweating when we are anxious – in the Stone Age a useful way of making our bodies slippery to elude an attacker, but less acceptable in today's world. Society is also to blame for making us feel we should conform to a certain body image – large breasts, small breasts and lopsided breasts are perfectly normal, but are included in this book because they can cause so much distress. Our genital organs and our sexual lives are never-ending sources of secret worries. And some embarrassments are very hard to explain – the baldness industry is worth millions, but baldness is a sign of male hormones so you might expect men to be more distressed by a full head of hair!

If your problem is not covered, let me know and we may well include it in the next edition.

Margaret Stearn

Write to:

Hatherleigh Press

5-22 46th Avenue Suite 200, Long Island City, NY 11101

Phone: 800-528-2550, E-mail: info@hatherleighpress.com

Talking to your doctor

Doctors know that many problems are difficult for their patients to discuss with them. If you feel anxious about discussing your problem with your doctor just remember:

- you will almost certainly not be the first person your doctor has encountered with this problem
- after their years of training, doctors are unshockable
- your doctor probably went into medicine in the first place because he/she wanted to help people (yes, really!); because your problem is distressing, he/she will gain a lot of satisfaction from resolving it.

Initiating the discussion

If you say something like, "I have a problem which I want to discuss with you, but I find it difficult to talk about," the doctor will immediately be on your side. Another possibility is to write a few lines about your problem, take the note with you to your appointment and ask the doctor to read it. Or take this book with you and use it as a starting point. Don't worry if talking makes you nervous or tearful – doctors are used to people being upset.

Confidentiality

You may be concerned about confidentiality. The best way of dealing with this is to ask the doctor. Say, "I have a rather embarrassing/personal problem which I want to discuss with you, but I am worried about confidentiality. How confidential is our discussion? Who will see the notes you make?"

What if you don't like your doctor?

You may dislike your doctor, or you may like him/her but feel he/she would be unsympathetic to this particular problem. If you genuinely don't like your doctor you should choose a new one. Some practices will let you change to another doctor within the practice, or will let you make all your appointments with other doctors within the practice without officially changing. Some practices don't allow this, so your only option if you don't like your doctor is to change to another practice.

If you like your doctor, but don't want to discuss this particular problem with him/her, simply say to the receptionist, "Just for this one appointment, I would like to see Dr Y instead of Dr X."

Health clinics

Visiting a health clinic
Health clinics deal with many genital and sexual problems, not just infections.

Why go to a clinic?
Staff at clinics are specially trained and experienced in genital problems; they also have a reputation for being kind and sympathetic and non-judgmental.

- As well as doctors and nurses, clinics usually have special counselors, called health advisers, who can help you with worries and give you additional information you may need.
- Clinics have facilities for doing tests for all genital infections. In many cases, they will be able to give you the results, and the treatment, straight away.
- You don't need a referral from your doctor to visit a clinic – simply call the clinic and make an appointment.
- Clinics are very confidential. They will ask if they can send the result of your tests to your doctor, but if you refuse they will not do so.

What sort of problems can a clinic help with?
You can attend a clinic for tests if you think you might have a sexually transmitted infection, even if you have no symptoms, or if you want an HIV test. Or you might have symptoms (such as a discharge). The clinic could help if you are worried about whether the appearance of your genitals is normal.

Finding the clinic
The telephone number is probably listed in the 'Business and Services' section of your phone book under 'Venereal Diseases' or 'Sexually Transmitted Diseases'. If not, telephone your local hospital and ask for information about the nearest clinic. When you telephone the clinic for an appointment, be sure to ask for clear directions. Clinics are often tucked away and difficult to find.

acne & pimples

- The worst ages for acne is 16–18 years for women and 18–19 years for men, but people of any age can get acne
- At 40 years of age, 5 women in 100 and 1 man in 100 have troublesome pimples or acne
- The ancient Egyptians relied on a pimple cream made from bulls' bile, ostrich egg, olive oil, salt and plant resin, mixed to a paste with flour and milk
- North Americans spend more than 2 billion dollars a year on acne treatments

How do pimples form?

The skin contains millions of sebaceous glands which secrete a grease, called sebum, through the skin pores onto the surface of the skin. Normally sebum simply helps to keep the skin healthy. A pimple forms when the pore becomes blocked by a plug of dead skin cells mixed with sebum. This usually happens because the sebaceous gland has produced more sebum than usual.

- A whitehead is a skin pore that is blocked by a plug deep down.
- A blackhead is a skin pore that has become plugged at its opening. The black color is a build up of the normal skin pigments from dead cells (the same pigment that is responsible for a suntan); it is not dirt.

The bacteria that normally live on the surface of the skin, called *Propionibacterium acnes,* move into the blocked pore behind the blackhead or whitehead. They may produce pus, leading to yellow pimples, and cause inflammation.

What is the difference between pimples and acne?

There is no real difference; it's just a matter of quantity. If you have a few, they are usually referred to as 'spots', 'pimples' or 'zits'. But if you have quite a lot of whiteheads, blackheads or angry-looking inflamed pores, it is referred to as *acne.*

Why do some people get acne?

No one knows why some people's skin secretes more sebum than others. However, the glands become particularly active soon after puberty, usually around the age of 11–14 years, and this is usually when pimples first develop.

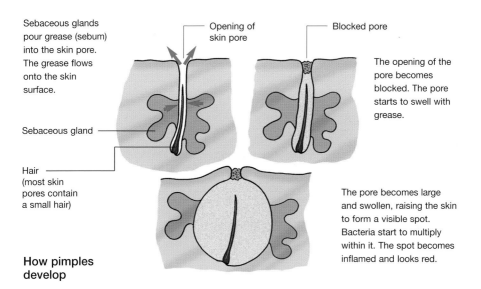

Sebaceous glands pour grease (sebum) into the skin pore. The grease flows onto the skin surface.

Sebaceous gland

Hair (most skin pores contain a small hair)

Opening of skin pore

Blocked pore

The opening of the pore becomes blocked. The pore starts to swell with grease.

The pore becomes large and swollen, raising the skin to form a visible spot. Bacteria start to multiply within it. The spot becomes inflamed and looks red.

How pimples develop

Some drugs can cause acne. The best-known examples are anabolic steroids taken by body-builders, but phenytoin (for epilepsy), rifampicin (for tuberculosis), vitamin B_{12} (for anemia) and lithium (for mood swings) can also produce acne. Occasionally, chemicals in the workplace, such as industrial oils, are responsible.

The female hormone called *estrogen* improves acne, whereas another female hormone, called *progesterone,* makes it worse. Most oral contraceptives contain both estrogen and progesterone, so it is not surprising that the pill worsens acne in some people and improves it in others. A progesterone-only pill would be a bad choice for someone with pimples.

Chefs and sauna masseurs find that their hot, humid environment worsens acne, though no one knows why exactly. Similarly, acne may worsen if you move to a hot country.

Improving your skin

Washing. Wash your face, neck and back twice a day with an unperfumed soap or a soap-free solution (the perfume in soaps, and soap itself, can irritate some skins). Don't wash more often than this or scrub your skin or use a harsh abrasive soap – you may dry the skin too much and make it oversensitive to acne treatments.

Acne: true or false?

Acne is caused by not washing properly – False

- Washing the skin is irrelevant to acne (except that overwashing can sometimes make the skin too sensitive to use anti-acne medications).

Stress worsens acne – Probably true

- For example, students often find their acne gets worse before exams. However, some experts think the reason is simply that when you are stressed you fiddle with your skin more.

Chocolate, sweets and fried foods make acne worse – False

- There is no scientific evidence for this.

Masturbation, too much sex or too little sex worsens acne – False

- These are total myths.

You can catch acne by skin contact, or by using the same flannel or towel as someone with acne – False

- Acne is not infectious.

Greasy hair hanging over the face causes spots – False

- The hair is greasy for the same reason that the pimples are present (which is overproduction of sebum).

Acne is worse premenstrually – True

- Many women notice their pimples are worse during the week before a period. Some women find acne improves during pregnancy, while others find that it gets worse.

Acne runs in families – True

- If either of your parents had acne, you are likely to have it.

Acne affects only the face, chest and back – False

- Although these are the most common sites, acne can affect any part of the body except the palms of the hands and the soles of the feet. It can sometimes occur on the arms, buttocks and legs as well as on the face, neck, back and chest.

Acne usually clears up on its own – True

- In 7 out of 10 people, acne will clear up on its own after 7 or 8 years. But there is no need to wait that long, as effective treatments are available.

Make-up. If you wear make-up, avoid heavy and greasy make-up; 'oil-free' make-up is available in some brands. Remove it at night with a gentle cleanser before washing. To disguise an individual pimple, use a blemish concealer stick; don't apply the stick to a large area or you may make the skin sensitive.

Squeezing. Discipline yourself not to squeeze or fiddle with your pimples, because this encourages scarring. For blackheads, you can buy a 'comedone spoon'. This is a tiny spoon with a hole in it, which you press onto the blackhead to release it from the pore; abandon the attempt if the blackhead doesn't come out easily. If you have a large yellow spot containing pus, which you feel you really must get rid of, pierce it with a needle and gently squeeze the pus out using a tissue. Wash your hands and sterilize the needle in a flame beforehand.

Pimple creams. Don't waste your money on anti-acne preparations which describe themselves as 'medicated'. Most of these have very little effect. They are also expensive, and you are likely to need to continue your anti-acne treatment for months or even years. Ask the pharmacist for 2.5% benzoyl peroxide cream or gel.

Before starting the cream or gel, draw a diagram of your face on a sheet of paper. Mark in the areas where your pimples are, and roughly how many. This will help you to decide whether the treatment works. Apply the treatment thinly twice a day after washing, avoiding the lips and eyes. After a week or two upgrade to the 5% and then the 10% strengths, unless you have excessive peeling and redness; some slight peeling is usual. If your skin feels very dry, buy an oil-free moisturizer (for example, Johnson's Clean and Clear).

After about 2 months, decide whether your pimple count has improved by about a third. If it has, continue with the benzoyl peroxide. You may need to continue it for several months. If there has not been improvement, see your doctor for some stronger treatment. You will also need to see your doctor if you have acne on your back – creams and lotions are difficult to apply to the back and tablet treatments might be more appropriate.

What your doctor can do

Most doctors are now sympathetic and helpful to people with pimples, and recognize how much psychological distress even mild acne can cause. Also, they have some effective treatments to offer, which was not the case a few years ago. Acne treatments usually control rather than cure the condition. This means that if you stop the treatment the acne often reappears.

Tretinoin. If blackheads and whiteheads are the main problem, tretinoin cream, lotion or gel is an effective treatment because it unblocks the pores by removing the build-up of dead skin cells. There is usually 60% improvement after 3 months' treatment. Some peeling and irritation of the skin often occurs. It can also make your skin sensitive to sunlight, so it should be applied at night and washed off in the morning, and you should use an oil-free sunscreen (at least SPF 15) during the day. Tretinoin should not be used by women who are pregnant or may become pregnant.

Adapalene is a new gel treatment, which your doctor might prescribe instead of tretinoin. Like tretinoin, it works for mild-to-moderate acne where there are blackheads and whiteheads. Its effectiveness is similar to tretinoin, (60% improvement after 3 months), but it needs to be applied only once a day (before bed).

Antibiotics. The doctor may suggest an antibiotic cream containing tetracycline, clindamycin or erythromycin. Some antibiotic creams also contain zinc, which enhances their action. For moderately severe acne, and especially if the pimples are inflamed and angry-looking, the usual treatment is antibiotic tablets (usually tetracyclines, but sometimes erythromycin). Unfortunately, to be effective, some tetracyclines have to be taken several times a day, which can be inconvenient. If you think this will be problematic for you, ask your doctor for a once-daily type of tetracycline (such as lymecycline, doxycycline or minocycline). Antibiotics have to be taken for at least 6 months; the acne will improve gradually over this period. Benzoyl peroxide should be used at the same time. The treatment may need to continue for 2 years.

Antibiotics can interfere with the contraceptive pill, so women need to use an additional method of contraception. Also, tetracyclines must not be taken during pregnancy, while breast-feeding or by children under 12, and some women develop thrush.

Hormonal treatment. Women have the option of using hormonal treatment for acne such as Dianette (ethinyloestradiol with cyproterone acetate). This is a contraceptive pill that blocks the action of the hormone called *testosterone*. Testosterone can encourage the overproduction of sebum; women, as well as men, normally have some testosterone circulating in their bodies.

Isotretinoin. For severe, lumpy acne the best treatment is isotretinoin tablets. For this your doctor will need to refer you to a dermatologist. This is usually very effective as it reduces sebum production, clears the build-up of the dead cells that block the pores and reduces inflammation. It is usually given for 4 months. Around half the people who use it are then permanently cured. In the other half, acne will reappear over the next 18 months. Isotretinoin has some side-effects, such as reddening and scaling of the skin, soreness of the lips and drying of the nose causing nosebleeds. The main problem is that it can cause abnormalities in a developing fetus, so women who might become pregnant must never take it, and contraception must be continued for a least a month after stopping it. If you start feeling depressed while taking it, see your doctor – in a few cases, isotretinoin has been linked to severe depression.

Burnt-out acne
Severe acne can leave scars. Though these will fade with time, if they are extensive but not too deep, and the acne is no longer flaring up, the dermatologist or your doctor can refer you to a plastic surgeon for dermabrasion. This is a relatively crude procedure in which the skin is 'planed down' using a high-speed wire brush. It can alter the pigmentation of the skin, so is not suitable for dark-skinned people. Acne scarring can also be treated with a laser, which removes the top layer of skin.

Dermabrasion and laser treatment are only effective for very shallow pitting of the skin. Scars which are deep and disfiguring can sometimes be cut out by a plastic surgeon. To lessen your chances of scars, try hard not to pick your pimples.

USEFUL CONTACTS
There are a host of acne-related sites on the Internet, most of them selling acne-related treatments. Use your judgment and talk to your doctor before purchasing any treatments.

There are also good books available. Try *The Good Skin Doctor: A Dematologist's Survival Guide to Acne* by Tony C. Chu and Anne Lovell. The book is published by Thorsons Publishing, and should be available at your local bookstore or on Amazon.com.

bad breath

- Many chemicals cause the smell in bad breath including hydrogen sulphide, methyl mercaptan and putrescine
- Garlic rubbed into the soles of the feet can be detected later in the breath
- "You can have affection for a murderer, but you cannot have an affection for a man whose breath stinks – habitually stinks, I mean." George Orwell, *The Road to Wigan Pier*

Most people worry about having bad breath or *halitosis*, as shown by the huge sales of breath fresheners. However, it is not easy to tell whether you have it or not. There is actually a psychological condition called *delusion of halitosis* or *halitophobia*, in which people have an unshakable belief that their breath smells, although in fact it does not. Their lives are totally dominated by their 'bad breath' and they are not amenable to reason. If you think that you have bad breath, it is worth finding out what the true situation is.

- If you find your gums bleed when you brush or floss your teeth it is almost certain that you have bad breath as well.
- Inspect your gums to see if they look red and swollen in places; if they do, it is likely you have bad breath.
- It is sometimes suggested that you can detect your own bad breath by breathing out through your mouth into a paper bag, and then breathing in rapidly from the bag through your nose. You might catch a whiff by this method, but usually it does not work because your nose is so used to your own breath smell.
- Put your tongue out as far as you can; lick your upper arm, or the inner surface of your wrist, wait 4 seconds and smell where you licked.
- If you are a smoker you probably have smoker's breath.
- Ask your dentist or dental hygienist; they are very used to being asked this question.
- Ask your partner or a close friend, though they may tell you unprompted!

How to clean your teeth

- Use a brush with a small head, about the size of a dime.

- Use only a pea-sized blob of toothpaste. Toothpaste is abrasive and too much can cause wear of the teeth.

- Clean two teeth at a time, using small circular or backward and forward movements (not up and down), counting to six for each pair.

- Aim the bristles towards the gum.

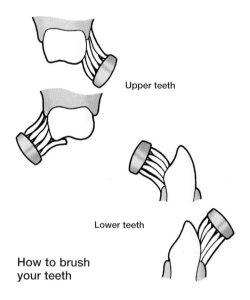

Upper teeth

Lower teeth

How to brush your teeth

'Morning breath'

Almost everyone has bad breath first thing in the morning. During the day, movement of the tongue and cheeks dislodges food debris and dead cells, and these are washed away by saliva. While we are asleep our tongue and cheeks do not move much, and the flow of saliva is reduced. The food residues stagnate in the mouth, and mouth bacteria rapidly break them down, releasing an unpleasant stale smell. Breathing through the mouth when sleeping tends to make this worse. Fortunately, morning breath normally disappears after breakfast or cleaning the teeth. Get your saliva going with a drink of water and lemon.

Temporary bad breath

Temporary bad breath is the lingering effect of cigarettes or of something you have eaten in the past 24–48 hours. Alcohol, onions, garlic, curries and other highly spiced foods, cured foods such as salamis, and smoked foods such as salmon are particularly likely to remain on the breath. The problem isn't simply that the smells stay in the mouth; these foods are digested and then broken down in the body, and the breakdown products of some – particularly alcohol, onions and garlic – are expelled in the breath for hours or days afterwards (this is the basis of the 'breathalyzer test' for alcohol).

Smoking also reduces the flow of saliva, which makes its smell linger even longer. Traditional remedies such as eating parsley help, and mouth fresheners disguise the smell. Clean your mouth by rinsing it thoroughly with warm water, giving it a good brushing with toothpaste and then rinsing thoroughly again.

Bad breath can even result from not eating. When no food is available, the body starts breaking down fat. Waste products from fat breakdown *(ketones)* are expelled in the breath, and smell like stale apples.

Persistent bad breath

Gum disease, according to dentists, is the usual cause of persistent bad breath. You will probably be unaware you have the problem because gum disease is not necessarily painful. The gum is likely to bleed when you brush your teeth. It will look very red, but goes pale for a moment if you press on it, and will be slightly swollen where it meets the teeth. Gum disease is caused by plaque, the sticky film of bacteria that naturally forms on the teeth of everyone every day. These bacteria tend to lodge between the teeth and where the teeth meet the gum. The waste products of the bacteria have a foul, stale smell. Apart from bad breath, gum disease can eventually cause loosening of the teeth.

Poor oral hygiene is an obvious cause. If you don't clean your teeth, you will soon develop bad breath.

A coated, furry tongue may or may not cause bad breath; dentists are still arguing about this one. Some say that bacteria, food particles and stagnant saliva builds up in the 'fur', particularly at the back of the tongue, and that everyone should brush the tongue with a toothbrush, or use a special tongue cleaner. Others say that brushing the tongue will make microscopic cracks in its surface, which will harbor bacteria and make the problem worse.

Chronic sinus infection can cause bad breath, particularly if there is *postnasal drip*. This is infected mucus that trickles down the back of the throat. It causes a ticklish cough, particularly when lying flat at night.

Gut problems used to be blamed, and enemas and laxatives were often given as cures, but in fact these have very little to do with bad breath. Your stomach is shut off from your throat and mouth by a tight ring of muscle at the base of the foodpipe, so it is normally a closed tube. Therefore no odor escapes from the stomach, except if you belch, or regurgitate food (vomit).

Anything that dries the mouth makes bad breath worse, because saliva cleanses the mouth. Tricyclic antidepressant drugs (such as amitriptyline) reduce saliva. Alcohol, alcohol-containing mouthwashes, heavy exercise and fasting can all result in a dry mouth and worsen a bad breath problem.

Isosorbide dinitrate, a drug for angina, sometimes produces an objectionable smell in the mouth.

What to do about persistent bad breath

A check-up by a dentist and a session with the dental hygienist is the first priority. Ask the dentist for a thorough cleaning and polish, and ask if there are any defects where plaque and food debris might be building up. Ask the hygienist to show you how to clean your teeth properly, and how to use floss to clean between the teeth. Give your teeth a thorough cleaning for 5 minutes (see page 17) at least once a day to remove the plaque, and use floss. Use a toothpick after meals to remove large food particles from between the teeth.

Brushing the tongue with a soft toothbrush once a day may be helpful. The most important part to clean is the back of the tongue, if you can do this without gagging. Do not overdo the brushing; the idea is to dislodge any bacteria and flush out stagnant saliva.

Chewing sugar-free gum can be helpful because it stimulates the flow of saliva and involves movements of the jaw and cheeks. Both these factors help to remove food debris and cleanse the mouth.

Mouthwashes, deodorizing mouth sprays or tablets will mask bad breath temporarily – useful after eating onion or garlic. Modern mouthwashes also contain antibacterial chemicals so, in theory, they should improve gum disease and mouth odor. There are six main types of mouthwash.
- A two-phase mouthwash which contains three antibacterial agents – natural essential oils, triclosan and cetylpyridinium. These absorb, lift and remove bacteria, debris, food

and dead cells which cause bad breath (see the result when you spit out). The oil phase absorbs smelly gases. The effect is said to last for 18 hours.

- Chlorhexidine gluconate is the most effective antibacterial wash, but tastes nasty and darkens teeth slightly for a few days.
- Phenolic mouthwashes (for example, Listerine) are almost as effective as chlorhexidine in reducing gum disease.
- Cetylpyridinium chloride is an effective antibacterial but it does not remain in the mouth for long after rinsing.
- Povidone-iodine (for example, Betadine) can cause irritation, and must not be used by pregnant women or children or for longer than 14 days.
- Chlorine dioxide rinses claim to eliminate the sulphur chemicals which are partly responsible for the bad smell of halitosis.

At present, most mouth rinses are acidic, and dentists worry that they might damage tooth enamel. There is also a possibility that the bacteria they eliminate could be replaced by more harmful types that can withstand the effects of mouthwashes.

Electric toothbrushes. Consider investing in an electric toothbrush. Some studies have shown that they remove plaque and reduce *gingivitis* (gum disease) better than a manual toothbrush.

USEFUL CONTACTS
American Dental Association
211 E. Chicago Ave.
Chicago, IL 60611
312/440-2500
Fax: 312/440-2800
www.ada.org

baldness

- It is normal to lose 50–100 hairs from the head each day
- Each hair on the head grows for about 5 years before being shed
- Eyebrow hairs grow for only 10 weeks
- Scalp hair grows at a rate of about 1 cm (just under $\frac{1}{2}$ an inch) a month
- We each have about 100,000 hairs on the scalp

How hair grows

The portion of the hair that we can see is called the shaft. Each shaft of hair protrudes from its follicle, which is a tube-like pouch just below the surface of the skin. The hair is attached to the base of the follicle by the hair root, which is where the hair actually grows and where it is nourished by blood capillaries.

Like the rest of the body, hairs are made of cells. As new cells form at its root, the hair is gradually pushed further and further out of the follicle. The cells at the base of each hair are close to the blood capillaries, and are living. As they get pushed further away from the base of the follicle they no longer have any nourishment, and so they die. As they die, they are transformed into a hard protein called keratin, which is also the material of which fingernails, toenails and animals' hooves and horns are made. So, each hair we see above the skin

Section through the skin showing hair

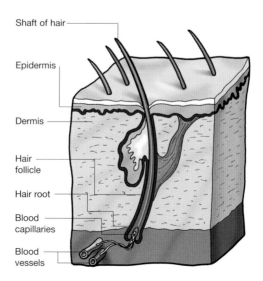

Shaft of hair

Epidermis

Dermis

Hair follicle

Hair root

Blood capillaries

Blood vessels

is dead protein. It is the follicle, which lies deep in the skin, that is the essential growing part of the hair.

Hair growth is not a continuous process: it has several stages.
- The first phase is the growing stage. Hair grows at about 1 cm each month, and this phase lasts for anything between 2 and 5 years.
- This is followed by a resting stage, during which there is no growth. This phase lasts for about 3 months, and is called *telogen*.
- At the end of the resting phase, the hair is shed, and the follicle starts to grow a new one.
- At any moment, 70–90% of the hair follicles of the scalp are growing hairs in the first phase; only 10–30% are in the resting phase.
- If a follicle is destroyed for any reason, no new hair will grow from it.

How baldness happens

If any of the stages of hair growth are disrupted, the individual may become bald. For example, if follicles shut down (meaning that they stay in the resting phase, and shed the hair) instead of growing new hairs, there will be less hair on the head. Another reason might be interference with the formation of new hair cells at the root during the growing phase; this occurs with some anti-cancer drugs. If follicles have been destroyed (as they might be by, for example, a burn, or by some skin diseases), there will be baldness in that area. An individual can also look bald if the hairs are growing but are so fragile that they break just as they emerge from the follicle.

In 1998, scientists at Columbia University in New York announced the discovery of a gene that appears to be the 'master switch' for hair growth. They found the gene after comparing the genes of hairless mice belonging to a mutant breed, and comparing those of 11 members of the same family who had lost all their hair. This discovery is a step towards understanding how the hair follicle works and how baldness happens, and may lead to effective treatments becoming available within a few years.

How to know if you are losing too much hair – the tug test

Bald areas are an obvious sign, but it can be difficult to tell whether your hair is getting thinner. Hold a small bunch of hair – about 15 or 20 hairs – between the thumb and index finger. Pull slowly and firmly. If more than six come out there may be a problem.

Male-pattern baldness

Receding hair is loss of hair at the sides of the forehead. It happens to most men eventually – usually at or after middle age, but it can start at any time after puberty. Some men also have loss of hair on top of the head, and eventually only the sides and back of the head have hair, forming a horseshoe shape. This is known as *common baldness, androgenic alopecia* or *male-pattern baldness.*

If you were able to look at the bald area under a microscope you would see that the hair follicles are shrunken, the hairs being produced are fine and short, and a higher proportion than usual of the follicles are in the resting phase.

Hair loss: true or false?

Some hairstyles can cause hair loss – True

- Styles that put tension on the hairs – such as tight ponytails, plaits or corn-rows – can cause loss of hair. Winding hair tightly onto rollers (especially heated rollers) can have the same damaging effect.

Brushing the hair 100 times a day will stimulate the circulation and prevent hair loss – False

- Vigorous brushing is more likely to injure the hairs and make the problem worse.

Hair needs to breathe, so wigs and toupees worsen loss of hair – False

- Hair does not need to breathe. Only the root of the hair is alive, and this gets its oxygen from the blood in the scalp. Wigs and hairpieces will only damage hair if they are too tight.

Frequent shampooing makes hair fall out – False

- The 50–100 hairs we lose each day often become tangled with the rest of the hair, but are washed out when we shampoo. So we see what seems like a lot of hair in the tub after shampooing, but in reality these hairs have been shed earlier.

Blow-drying and heated brushes can worsen hair loss – True

- The reason is that extreme heat damages the proteins in the hairs, making them fragile and liable to break off. Brushing the hair during blow-drying causes more damage. Careless use of heated brushes can even burn the scalp, so that the hair follicles are permanently damaged in that area.

Protein-containing conditioners and shampoos nourish the hair and help it to grow – False

- Protein-containing conditioners only temporarily fill in defects on the surface of the hair shaft, making it smoother and thicker.

Measuring baldness in men – the Norwood-Hamilton scale is used to classify the type and stage of common baldness in men

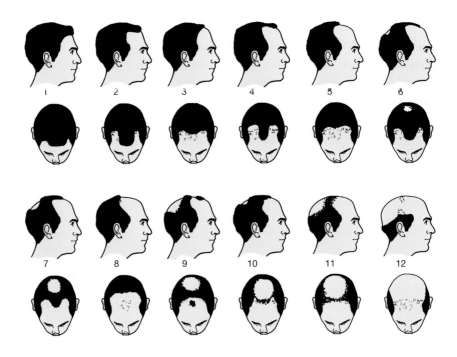

Adapted from Norwood O T and Schiell R D, *Hair Transplant Surgery*. 2nd edn. 1984. Courtesy of Charles C Thomas, Publisher Ltd., Springfield, Illinois, USA.

Three factors are at work in male-pattern baldness: male hormones, heredity (genetics) and aging.

Maleness was recognized by Aristotle as a cause of baldness. He wrote that "no boy, woman or castrated male ever becomes bald" and he thought that baldness was a sign of virility (he was bald himself!). To a large degree, science has proved him right. Baldness is the result of hair follicles reacting to male hormones. However, men with male-pattern baldness don't have higher levels of male hormones than other men. It is simply that their hair follicles respond to the hormones differently.

The main male hormone is testosterone. Both men and women have testosterone in the blood, but men have higher levels. The skin of the scalp converts testosterone to another substance called *dihydrotestosterone* (DHT). Hair follicles in areas that are destined to become bald seem to be especially sensitive to DHT, and shrink when exposed to it. Follicles on the sides and back of the head are not affected by DHT.

Heredity (genetics) is important. If you have relatives with thin hair or who are bald, you may well develop the same problem. This tendency can be inherited from either the mother's or the father's side of the family (but the mother herself would usually be unaffected, or her hair might start thinning after the menopause). Inheritance probably makes the follicles extra sensitive to DHT.

Aging makes baldness more likely. Forty per cent of men have noticeable hair loss by age 35, and 65% by age 60. Most elderly people have thin, fine hair even if they are not noticeably bald.

Treatments that don't work

The most popular medical book of our great-grandparents' day, *The Household Physician,* advised that baldness could be prevented by "quickening the circulation in the scalp, such as by washing the head every morning in cold water, then drying with a rough towel by vigorous rubbing, and brushing with a hard brush until the scalp becomes red." Others recommended rubbing in onion juice or curry paste with a stiff brush to irritate the scalp. In fact, lack of circulation is not the problem in baldness and these measures would make the problem worse by damaging the hairs. Similarly, hanging upside down to improve the circulation in the scalp will not produce any improvement.

It used to be thought that excess grease on the scalp caused hair loss, and male-pattern baldness was called *seborrhoeic* (greasy) *baldness*. In fact, bald areas appear greasy only because there is no hair to take up the grease; the actual amount of grease being produced is normal. Some baldness 'cures' claim to act by reducing grease; they make no difference. Removing grease makes hair look more fluffy, but doesn't actually increase the amount of hair.

Treatments that work

- Keeping existing hair and scalp healthy makes obvious sense.
- Wash your hair once or twice a week with a mild shampoo; dirty hair lies flatter and looks more sparse.
- Avoid anything that could make the hairs liable to break. For example, after washing

don't rub your hair vigorously or use a hot hairdryer. Instead, pat it dry with a soft towel or use a low setting on the dryer or, even better, let it dry naturally. Use a brush with soft bristles. Undo any tangles with your fingers, rather than pulling with a comb.

- Protect bald areas from sun damage. Scalp Bloc has been specially prepared for this purpose, and is available from pharmacies. It is non-scented and non-greasy.

Rogaine (minoxidil) lotion stimulates hair growth in balding areas. It works by keeping hair follicles in the growth phase for longer, giving bigger hairs. No effect is seen for the first 3 or 4 months. Unfortunately it is not successful for everyone – only about 35% of men have some regrowth of hair, and this is often fine and downy – and the manufacturers advise users to give up if there has been no regrowth after using it for a year.

It has to be applied religiously twice a day, 7 days a week and does not produce a permanent cure. If the treatment is stopped, the follicles go back to how they would have been without Rogaine.

Rogaine 2% lotion can be bought from pharmacies without a prescription. It appears to stabilize hair growth in about 80% of men and seems to be safe, but it is important to read the manufacturer's leaflet. For example, it should probably not be used by people taking drugs for blood pressure, or who have angina. The solution contains alcohol, and can cause irritation in some people. The main problem is the cost – around $40 for a month's treatment. This means that you have to spend $250 before seeing any benefit. If you continue for a year and then give up because it has not had any effect, you will have spent $450 for nothing.

Rogaine 5% lotion is probably more effective, but cannot be bought without a private prescription.

Hair transplantation is a surgical procedure, based on the fact that hair follicles from the sides and back of the head will continue to grow, even when transplanted to bald areas. In the past, small plugs of skin less than half a centimeter across and containing about 100 hair follicles, were transplanted. These 'plug grafts' were not very successful, because they gave an unnatural 'tufted' appearance, like doll's hair, but are still sometimes used to give coverage in the middle of large areas.

Surgeons are now able to transplant much smaller grafts.

- Minigrafts (3–4 hairs/graft) are commonly used for men who are thinning over a large area, to fill in gaps around plug grafts.

- Micrografts (1–2 hairs/graft) are often used along hairlines especially if the hairline has receded only slightly.
- Unigrafts (1 hair/graft) look very natural and so are used along the frontal hairline, or for areas that are thinning but not yet bald. They are also suitable for men who have a large bald area and would be satisfied with a light but natural-looking thin coverage.

After a local anesthetic injection, a small piece of skin is removed from an area where there is still plenty of hair and where it will not show, such as the back of the head, just above the neck (the 'donor site'). The surgeon cuts out the tiny grafts from this piece of skin, and then places them into tiny incisions in the bald area. In the case of unigrafts, the hole to receive the graft is simply made with a needle. The grafts do not need any stitches; they are held in place by the clotting action of the blood. The donor site and the grafts heal very quickly, because the scalp has a very good blood supply.

Usually, an individual will need 300–700 grafts, but of course this depends on the size of the bald area. About 100 are done at each session, which takes about 3 hours. The hair can usually be washed the next day. After a few months it is often difficult to distinguish between the grafts and the areas of normal hair.

The main disadvantage of hair transplantation is that the procedure is drawn out and costly. Also, many men are dissatisfied with the result. This may be partly because expectations are too high. It also depends on the skill of the surgeon. Choose a reputable practice and have a detailed preliminary discussion so that you know what the result will be. Find out how many sessions you will need, what coverage you will achieve and precisely what the total cost will be.

You should also ask what possible problems might occur. For example:

- As with any surgical procedure, there is a risk of infection of the skin
- The new grafts may not grow properly (and if this happens, nothing can be done)
- The transplanted hair may be a slightly different color from the surrounding hair, but this can be disguised by a dye if necessary
- Scarring or a lumpy appearance known as 'cobblestoning' may occur, but is unlikely with the modern small grafts.

If you have tight curly hair, you need a particularly detailed discussion with the surgeon, because hair transplantation could be problematic. Firstly, the hair follicles are curled, so it is more difficult for the surgeon to prepare the tiny grafts; they may be damaged and not grow well. Secondly, each graft may develop an unsightly lumpy scar, so the surgeon should do an initial test by transplanting just two or three to an inconspicuous area.

Scalp reduction (scalp excision) is a surgical operation in which the hairless portion of the scalp is pulled up tightly and the excess removed surgically, so that the area that has no hair is reduced. It is best for older men whose scalps are looser. There will be a scar from the incision, but this will fade in time. The result can sometimes look odd, because the remaining hair may be pulled up to an unnatural position. The advantage is that it is usually a 'one-off' procedure, unlike hair transplantation.

Finasteride (Propecia) is a drug for an enlarged prostate gland. It works by preventing testosterone from being converted into DHT (see pages 24–25), so in theory it might prevent or improve male-pattern baldness. It has to be taken constantly. Because it is a tablet rather than a lotion it is more convenient than Rogaine, and it seems to be as effective or better than Rogaine.

The most worrying problem with finasteride is that, in a pregnant woman, it can interfere with development of the genitals if the baby in her womb is male. This means that a woman who is pregnant or who could become pregnant should not even handle the tablets. When a man is taking finasteride there will be some in his semen, and during intercourse this will be transferred to the woman. This means that a couple should not try to conceive if the man is taking the drug.

Finasteride: effectiveness and problems

In a study, 945 men with male-pattern baldness took 1 mg finasteride and 600 similar men were given placebos and acted as a comparison group. The results of the study were reported at the 1997 Annual Meeting of the American Academy of Dermatology and were as follows:

- 65% of men who received finasteride had some hair growth
- on average, a one-inch diameter bald patch grew 107 extra hairs
- not much improvement occurred before 3 months
- 1.8% reported decreased sexual desire (but so did 1.3% given the dummy tablets)
- 1.3% reported difficulty in achieving an erection (but so did 0.7% given the dummy tablets)
- 0.8% reported a decrease in the amount of semen (but so did 0.4% given the dummy tablets)

Bald patches

Alopecia areata. Baldness which is in patches, and not in the typical male pattern is usually *alopecia areata*. This occurs in about 3% of people and affects men and women equally. It can occur at any age, but in most people it occurs between the ages of 5 and 40 years. The cause is not known, although it is slightly more common in people with thyroid disease.

The hair is lost completely from the patch, leaving a smooth, shiny scalp. A magnifying glass shows that the openings of the hair follicles are still present, but there are no hairs protruding from them. There may be short, distorted hairs at the edge of the bald patch. There may be only one patch, or there may be several. Sometimes there is a more diffuse 'moth-eaten' appearance, rather than distinct patches.

Alopecia areata can be very distressing, but the good news is that the hair follicles are not permanently damaged so regrowth of hair usually occurs. Regrowth is unpredictable, but usually occurs in 6–9 months. At first the new hair may be white, but after 12–18 months the color returns to normal. In some people the problem recurs after a few years.

In a few people, regrowth can be temporarily encouraged with Rogaine solution but the effect lasts only while the lotion is being used. Some doctors inject steroids into the scalp or prescribe steroid creams, but these only occasionally result in some regrowth. Dithranol is a cream or paste made from tar, and is used mainly to treat the skin disease psoriasis. In some people it produces some regrowth of hair. It is rubbed into the scalp and washed off after a few hours. Dithranol is messy, and stains clothing.

Hair pulling. Children quite commonly develop a habit of pulling the hair; there will be a patch of hair loss with stubbly regrowth. Adults (especially women) can develop a similar habit which can be very persistent and have a psychological basis. Hair can also be pulled out patchily by tight ponytails or corn-row styles.

Total baldness

Hair loss is a side-effect of some chemotherapy treatments for cancer. Although this is upsetting, at least the sufferer is prepared for it and knows the hair will regrow after the chemotherapy is over.

Suddenly losing all your scalp hair out of the blue, for no apparent reason, is a frightening and distressing experience. It can happen to both men and women. Elizabeth Steel, who has written a book about her experience, says, "When you suddenly lose all your hair as an adult, you feel immediately humiliated. It destroys your confidence in yourself in every aspect of your life. When your hair goes and self-esteem with it, your self-image is shattered."

This condition is called *alopecia totalis*. If it affects the body hair as well as the scalp hair (eyelashes, pubic hair) it is known as *alopecia universalis*. However, the fact that it has a name doesn't mean that it is understood. In most cases it is a mystery, but the follicles are not destroyed so regrowth is always a possibility. It may start as a small bald patch of alopecia areata which extends over a few months until there is no hair left, or all the hair may fall out over just a day or two. Regrowth can occur, but is not as likely as in the smaller patches of alopecia areata.

What your doctor can do. Your doctor should refer you to a dermatologist, who may try some of the following treatments. Unfortunately, the results of the treatments are very unpredictable.

- Rogaine may produce regrowth of hair but, as in male-pattern baldness, it may take several months before any effect is seen and the new hair will start to fall out after the treatment is stopped.
- Injecting steroids into the scalp is not suitable for the large area of total baldness, but steroid creams produce slight regrowth in some cases.
- Dithranol, as in patchy alopecia, sometimes produces some regrowth but it is often scanty.
- PUVA therapy is long-wave ultraviolet light. It is painless. It produces regrowth in up to 50% of people, and often works for people who have not responded to any other treatments. However, when the treatment is stopped only a few are cured. This means that the treatment has to be continued, which has two disadvantages. Firstly, it is time-consuming because between two and five sessions per week are needed. Secondly, like sunlight, it causes aging of the skin and the risk of skin cancers.
- Immunotherapy is based on the idea that in alopecia the hair follicles are attacked by the body's own immune system. The treatment involves making the scalp sensitive to a chemical and then repeatedly applying the chemical. Some doctors believe this works by turning the immune system away from attacking the hair follicle, by making it attack the chemical instead. The chemicals used most often are dinitrochlorbenzene, squaric acid dibutylester and diphencyprone. This technique results in hair growth in 30–40% of people, but the treatment has to be

given weekly for many months. The result may not be permanent, but usually lasts for at least 6 months.

- New therapies are being researched. For example, a damaging substance called tumour necrosis factor has been found in the hair follicles in alopecia, so treatment with antibodies to tumour necrosis factor is a future possibility.

What you can do. The main task of anyone with alopecia totalis or alopecia universalis is a psychological one, and it is not easy. It involves working out a way of living with the condition, and for this, Hairline International, the patients' society founded by Elizabeth Steel (see Useful Contacts), is a great help. It is important to remember that the hair follicles are not destroyed, so hair growth can occur at any time, even after many years. Elizabeth herself now has a full head of hair.

Thinning hair

If you think your hair is thinning, it is important to check that this is actually the case. Try the tug test (see page 22), and remember that it is normal to lose 50–100 hairs a day. Sometimes thinning of the hair can be entirely in the mind, as a symptom of depression. Thinning of hair all over the scalp (rather than patchy baldness) can be due to various causes. In the case of mental or physical stress, it often occurs 2–3 months after the event. This is because at the time of the stress many follicles enter telogen (the resting phase) prematurely, and are then shed together at the end of telogen a few months later. In this situation the hair loss usually recovers completely.

If you believe your hair is thinning, do not assume it is due to stress. See your doctor, who will be able to exclude the common causes (such as thyroid deficiency and iron deficiency). Many drugs – not just those in the table on page 32 – can cause hair loss, and the doctor will be able to check if this is a possibility.

Often no cause can be found. In some of these cases the hair will recover in time, but in others it remains thin.

It is important to keep thinning hair as healthy as possible, so the general recommendations for looking after hair (see page 25) apply. If there is no curable cause, and the thinning is distressing, it may be worth trying Rogaine. Bear in mind that Rogaine will take several months to show any effect, and works in only a proportion of cases.

Hair loss in women

In the words of Elizabeth Steel, hair loss is "miserable enough for a man: a downright catastrophe for a woman." A survey by Hairline International, the baldness support group, found that 78% of its female members no longer felt like women, 40% said their marriage had suffered and 63% had considered suicide.

Women who lose hair often worry that they are going bald like a man, and that their hormones are becoming masculinized. In fact patchy baldness (alopecia areata) and total baldness (alopecia totalis and alopecia universalis) are unrelated to hormones and occur equally commonly in men and women.

Like men, women develop widening partings and thinning of the hair all over the scalp, with age; this is normal. Hair can also become thin at the front, similar to the male pattern. This is simply because the hair follicles are responding in exactly the same way as in balding men to the testosterone in the blood. All women have testosterone; this is perfectly normal. The balding does not mean that the woman has high levels; it simply means that the hair follicles on her scalp are over-sensitive, probably inherited. Total baldness is very unlikely in this situation and in up to 50% of cases, Rogaine will produce some improvement.

In a few cases women develop male-pattern baldness with other male characteristics such as growth of hair on the face, deepening of the voice and menstrual disturbance. This can mean that too much testosterone is being produced by a tumor, so it is important to see the doctor so that appropriate tests can be done.

Causes of thinning hair
- **Age:** most old people have thinner hair than when they were young.
- **Heredity:** some people are programmed to have thin hair, particularly as they get older.
- **Hormone disorders,** particularly underactive thyroid gland.
- **Drugs** such as anti-cancer drugs, allopurinol (used for gout), chloroquine (antimalarial).
- **Iron deficiency** (most likely in women who are vegetarians).
- **Severe mental stress,** such as bereavement.
- **Severe physical illness** of any sort, but particularly a high fever or severe infection – the hair grows again on recovery.
- **Childbirth:** it is common to shed a lot of hair for 1–6 months after childbirth, but this usually grows again afterwards.
- **The connective tissue disease** systemic lupus erythematosus (SLE).

Wigs and hairpieces

Most people with extensive hair loss – usually caused by alopecia totalis or cancer chemotherapy – prefer to wear a wig. In recent years wigs have improved greatly, and it is no longer painfully obvious that someone is wearing one.

Your insurance company may supply wigs if the doctor (usually a dermatologist) considers it necessary. The wigs are lightweight acrylic and look extremely natural. They can be washed, and it does not matter if they are rained on. Because they are in stock sizes they can be obtained quickly. Most people have two – one to wear and one to wash. For totally bald heads, special wig tape is available to stop the wig slipping.

Some people still prefer a real hair wig, but these are more expensive even when you have insurance. They are made to measure, taking 6–8 weeks. They cannot be washed, and must be protected from rain. They are also more trouble than an acrylic wig, because they have to be styled and set like real hair. Professional cleaning costs about $15.

In her useful book *Hair Loss,* Elizabeth Steel makes the following points about wigs:

- If you decide to buy your wig privately from a department store, explain your predicament and ask for a private fitting room.
- You will probably feel you look very odd in the first few wigs you try on – partly because you haven't seen yourself with hair for a while. Persevere until you find one you like. Remember, even a new haircut can take time to get used to.
- Each time, make sure you put the wig on properly – it is quite easy to put a wig on backwards. (The tapes to adjust the size will be at the back.)
- At home, don't leave your wigs lying around.
- If you feel happier going to bed in your wig, do so.
- Remember that at a party you will not be the only one wearing something false. What about false nails, bosoms and teeth?

For male-pattern baldness, some men like to wear a hairpiece. Like wigs, these have improved in recent years and some now look very natural, if carefully matched to the existing hair. Some clinics suggest implanting clips into the scalp to hold the hairpiece more firmly in place, but this is not to be recommended because it can result in inflammation and infection of the scalp.

Clinics also offer implantation of artificial hair, which has the same strength, thickness and color as natural hair. Each 'hair' is inserted individually by an injection technique. This is also not to be recommended, because the scalp never gets used to the foreign material and there is always a risk of infection, and rejection with inflammation. Although the result may look good to start with, in time the hairs will break.

USEFUL CONTACTS

The American Cancer Society (www.cancer.org) has a program called "Look Good...Feel Better." This is a community based, free national service which teaches female cancer patients beauty techniques to help enhance their appearance and self-image during chemotherapy and radiation treatments

Hair Loss: Coping with Alopecia Areata and Thinning Hair by Elizabeth Steel (Harper Collins) is a practical guide to coping with different types of hair loss.

The Bald Truth: The First Complete Guide to Preventing and Treating Hair Loss by Spencer David Kobren, Diance B. Eisman (Foreword), Eugene H. Eisman and David Kobren (Pocket Books) is a practical guide to male pattern baldness.

belly button
discharge

The belly button can easily become infected by *Candida*, or other fungi – it is just the sort of warm, moist crevice that fungi like. If you have a fungal infection the belly button will look red, and the redness may extend to the surrounding skin for a few millimeters. It may be itchy.

Bacteria may also infect the belly button, often taking advantage of the damage already done by the fungi. This leads to scabbing and a yellowish discharge.

Redness may not be an infection at all – it may be caused by *psoriasis,* a skin disorder. On the arms and legs psoriasis causes scaly patches, but in moist areas like the belly button there is no scaliness – it just looks red and shiny. Usually, but not always, you will have psoriasis somewhere else on your body.

What to do
- Resist the urge to pick or scratch.
- Don't try to turn your belly button inside-out to clean it properly – just wash it gently using water to which you have added enough salt to give it a salty taste (about a tablespoonful in a bowl, or two handfuls in the bath). If you have a shower, use the shower head to rinse it well. Carefully dab it dry.
- Don't dab on any antiseptics, or add antiseptic to your bath water. This could irritate the skin and make it worse.
- Stop applying any creams from the chemist – they could be making it worse.
- If it doesn't start improving within a few days, or there is a yellowish discharge, see your doctor. You may need an antibiotic cream.

blushing

Blushing of the cheeks and nose (and sometimes the forehead and chin) is a normal emotional response. This is why it is annoying and can be embarrassing. Without our permission, our body is giving away emotions that we may prefer to keep secret; we may not want the world to know that we feel anxious or excited. Flushing and blushing are two words for the same thing – flushing is the word used by doctors.

Blushing caused by anxiety

There is no magic drug to prevent the normal blushing caused by anxiety. The best approaches are:

- Deciding not to mind it
- Controlling the anxiety by other means.

Bear in mind that your face is probably not as red as you think it is. Does it really matter if other people know that you are nervous? Everyone knows that giving a speech, meeting new people, asking someone out, being complimented or having an argument (or any other situation that makes you blush) are circumstances that make everyone nervous – whether or not they are prone to blushing.

If you think that you tend to be over-fearful or apprehensive, relaxation therapy or cognitive therapy (which helps you to see situations in a different light) may help. Your doctor will be able to give you advice about these.

If your blushing is so bad that it is really affecting your life, ask your doctor about an *endoscopic transthoracic sympathectomy* operation. This destroys the nerves that dilate the tiny blood vessels in the face. It is a relatively new treatment for blushing and, like any operation, has some risks. A survey of 224 patients, 8 months after this operation, suggested that 85% were pleased with the result.

Blushing caused by drugs

A few drugs can cause blushing, check whether you are taking any of the following:

- chlorpropamide can cause flushing if you take it with alcohol

- glyceryl trinitrate, isosorbide dinitrate
- tamoxifen
- buserelin, goserelin, leuprorelin, triptorelin.

Blushing at menopause

Most women experience blushes around menopause. They can be the earliest sign, so you can have them while your periods are still quite regular. In fact, a survey showed that 41% of women whose periods were still regular, but who were over the age of 39, blushed frequently. This usually goes on for 2–3 years, but 1 in 4 women has this for 5 years, and an unlucky 1 in 20 has it for the rest of her life.

A menopausal blush is an unpleasant sensation of heat which begins in the face, head or chest. Often, there is sweating and visible redness of the skin. It usually passes after a minute or two, leaving a feeling of coldness. Some women have just the flush without the sweating, while others sweat profusely but hardly flush. Flushes may occur frequently, even several times an hour, or just occasionally. Some women find that any slightly stressful situation will bring on a blush, or that they are more likely to happen when they are warm (for example, in bed, in an over-heated room, on vacation in a warm place). The flushes and sweats disturb sleep – some women wake covered in sweat – and this results in lethargy and irritability during the day.

You can help yourself by:

- Cutting down on alcohol and coffee, which tend to provoke flushes
- Avoiding spicy foods
- Keeping cool – wear several layers of light clothing, instead of one thick item, so you can easily peel something off
- Wearing a cotton bra (such as a sports bra) instead of a nylon one – the cotton will absorb sweat
- Taking a shower instead of a bath to cool down.

Plant estrogens. Some fruits and vegetables contain estrogen-like substances known as *phytoestrogens* (see table overleaf). Bacteria in the stomach can convert these into estrogens that the body can use. In theory, eating these foods should help menopausal symptoms like blushing. Japanese women, whose diets are packed with phytoestrogens, particularly soya, have less menopausal discomfort than women of other cultures.

The only problem with phytoestrogens is that they are 100–10,000-times weaker than human estrogens. You would have to consume a huge amount of these foods before the phytoestrogens could have any effect on really troublesome blushing, but you might find that they help a bit. A study of soya protein as a possible treatment for hot flushes was reported at the 1997 American Heart Meeting; the soya made the flushes less severe, but did not reduce the number of times that they happened. The easiest way to take soya is to add a pint of soya milk to your daily diet, or to switch to a soya bread, which is available from supermarkets.

Health shops and homeopathic pharmacies sell various remedies for hot flushes. Some of these, such as dong quai (Chinese angelica), licorice root and black cohosh, contain phytoestrogens. Others contain bizarre ingredients, such as cuttlefish ink (sepia), pulsatilla, graphites, snake venoms or sulphur. There is little scientific evidence to back up the manufacturers' claims that these remedies are effective.

Hormone replacement therapy (HRT) is the most effective treatment for menopausal flushing. This consists of estrogen and (unless you had a hysterectomy) a daily dose of progesterone for 14 days of the month. In some women the flushes stop immediately as soon as they start HRT, but usually they gradually decrease over 3 months.

Foods that contain phytoestrogens

● alfalfa	● parsley
● apples	● peas
● barley	● pomegranates
● carrots	● potatoes
● cherries	● red beans
● dates	● rice
● fennel	● rye
● French beans	● sage
● garlic	● sesame
● green beans	● soybeans
● licorice	● tofu
● oats	● wheat

Doctors are still arguing about how long women should stay on HRT. You might imagine that when you stop taking HRT the falling levels of hormones will make the flushes reappear. This does sometimes happen, but not in all women. When you stop HRT, the dose can be reduced very gradually so that the body becomes used to the falling levels, whereas during the natural menopause the hormone levels can go up and down like a rollercoaster.

bottoms

Painful anus

"I dread having to go to the bathroom, because it's so painful"

Anal pain isn't always due to hemorrhoids; there are a number of other quite common causes.

A knife-like pain when you have your bowels open, which may last for 10–15 minutes afterwards, is probably caused by an *anal fissure*. You may notice some bright red blood on the toilet paper at the same time. An anal fissure is a split in the anal skin, just inside the anus, usually towards the back. You may be able to feel a small lump alongside the crack; this is a *skin tag*. Anal fissures are most common in teenagers and young adults, and there has often been a period of constipation beforehand. They can heal on their own, but it takes a long time and the scar often splits again.

If you think you have a fissure, smear some painkilling gel around the area just before you have your bowels open. This prevents the anus going into a spasm, which can make the problem worse. Don't use the gel at any other time, or for more than a week, because you can easily develop an allergy to its ingredients. If you notice soreness and itching, as well as the sharp pain, it is quite likely that the gel is responsible. It is also important to avoid becoming constipated – eat lots of bran cereals, fruit and vegetables.

If the problem persists for more than 14 days, your doctor can send you to the rectal clinic at your local hospital. Until recently, the usual treatment was a small operation under a general anesthetic. This operation overcomes the spasm of the anal muscle but, though the pain relief is dramatic and instantaneous, it may leave you less able to control wind.

Instead of an operation, two new treatments are being tried out in some hospitals. One uses glyceryl trinitrate ointment, which is applied several times a day for 6 weeks. This seems to heal 60–70% of cases. The other treatment is an injection of botulinum toxin into the muscle of the anus.

A similar pain can be caused by herpes simplex virus, which can infect the anal area in both homosexuals and heterosexuals. At the anus, herpes often forms a crack rather than the small ulcers that tend to occur elsewhere. The soreness occurs in episodes, each lasting for a few days. A clinic (see page 9) will be able to take a swab to check for the virus if you visit the clinic as soon as an episode starts.

A nagging, aching discomfort made worse by defecation could be due to hemorrhoids (see page 119).

A throbbing pain, worsening over a few days, and bad enough to disturb your sleep, is likely to be caused by an abcess. You may be able to feel a tender swelling in the skin close to the anus, or the abcess may be hidden inside. This is unlikely to go away on its own; it needs to be lanced by a doctor, so see your doctor for this simple procedure.

An occasional, severe, cramp-like pain deep in the anal canal, lasting about half an hour is probably a condition called *proctalgia fugax*. It is a mysterious condition, and usually affects middle-aged men; no one knows what causes it. The pain often wakes sufferers at night, and men may have an erection at the same time. The pain goes away of its own accord, and there are no other effects. The best treatment is to take 2 paracetamols and a hot drink, and hope that it won't happen again.

A continuous aching pain in the anus needs to be sorted out by your doctor. It is most often caused by a back problem (when a part of the spine presses on a nerve).

Anal itching

"My anus is so itchy, I can't stop scratching"

Anal itching can be just an annoyance, or can be so troublesome that it dominates your life. It is usually made worse by warmth, and is often most troublesome in bed. The skin round the anus easily becomes irritated and inflamed. This is because it is difficult to keep the area clean and dry; the skin is crinkly and traps tiny fecal particles. It is also sweaty and airless, and it may be moist from an anal or vaginal discharge. When the anus becomes irritated, scratching is a natural reaction, but this damages the skin further. Ointments and creams can cause further problems by keeping the area damp.

Causes of anal itching

Poor hygiene is probably the most common reason.

Hemorrhoids can be very itchy, partly because of the slimy discharge they produce (see page 119).

Threadworms are tiny worms, about 13 mm long, that live in the lower part of the bowel. The female worms creep out of the anus at night, and lay their eggs on the skin. This causes intense itching at night. When you scratch, the eggs lodge under your fingernails, and it is easy to transfer them to your mouth and re-infect yourself.

Fungal infections – similar to thrush or athlete's foot – are another common cause. Fungi love warm, damp and damaged skin, so if you have an itchy anus for any reason and then damage the skin by scratching, fungi can take hold and make it worse.

Sexually transmitted infections are what most people worry about, but are not usually the reason. Genital warts (caused by papillomavirus) thrive in warm, moist conditions such as the skin near the anus and can be very itchy. Genital herpes (caused by herpes virus) can also infect the anus, and causes itching just before the sores appear and also during the healing stage. Both these viruses can occur round the anus in heterosexuals as well as homosexuals. The anus may be the only site of infection; the fact that you don't have genital warts or herpes elsewhere doesn't rule them out.

Skin conditions, such as psoriasis or eczema, can affect the skin around the anus.

Ointments and creams are notorious causes of anal itching. If you have itching, it is a natural reaction to buy an anesthetic gel for the anal area. Most of these are labelled 'for hemorrhoids' and contain lignocaine or benzocaine with other ingredients. At first they help, but then the itching returns because you become sensitive to one of the ingredients in the cream or ointment and they are keeping the area moist. They should never be used for more than a week at a time.

Pre-moistened toilet tissues (wipes) sometimes contain a preservative called Euxyl K 400. This contains two chemicals, one of which, methyldibromoglutaronitrile, often causes a skin allergy. If you develop anal itching after using pre-moistened wipes, this could be the cause.

Sensitivities and allergies to other chemicals – such as bubble baths and perfumed soaps – may be responsible.

Tetracycline, an antibiotic, commonly causes anal itching.

Anxiety tends to make the brain hyper-alert to body feelings that we may otherwise be able to ignore, so if you are going through an anxious period a symptom such as itching can become magnified.

Pleasure: it is worth asking yourself whether you are deriving a perverse, almost erotic, pain/pleasure from scratching the itchy area, which is keeping the irritation going.

You can help yourself by:
- Washing the anal area after you have opened your bowels. Avoid rubbing with rough toilet paper or bars of soap; soap left in the skin creases can be irritating so rinse well. Dab gently with a soft towel to dry – don't rub – or use a hairdryer.
- Keeping a cotton wool ball, dusted with powder, against the anus, inside your pants or knickers. Use baby powder (not perfumed talcum powder) to dust it or, even better, special drying powder from the pharmacist. Change it each time you wash.
- Wearing cotton underwear. Avoid tights, because they encourage sweating and moistness in the anal area. Avoid anything that keeps the buttocks close together.
- Not using biological washing powders or perfumed fabric softeners when washing your underwear. Instead, use a detergent labelled 'for sensitive skin'.
- Never scratching.
- Not using any steroid creams or anesthetic creams or greasy creams (such as Vaseline) on the area; greasy creams keep the skin soggy and make the problem worse.
- Using carbolic lotion. Buy it (1 in 100 strength) from the pharmacist, and dab it on with cotton wool, twice a day.
- Feeling round the anus for lumps. This may not be easy, because the skin round the anus is normally puckered. A lump might be a wart (see page 77), a hemorrhoid (see page 119) or a skin tag alongside an anal fissure (see page 40).

Your doctor can check to see whether you have any conditions such as hemorrhoids, anal fissure, warts, psoriasis, eczema, fungal infections or other infections that need treatment.

Threadworms can be eliminated with mebendazole. The other members of your household will also need to be treated. Wash your hands and scrub your nails before eating and after each visit to the toilet, and wash the anal area in the morning to get rid of any eggs deposited during the night.

breasts

Lopsided breasts

One in twenty women has one breast bigger than the other – just as it is common to have one foot bigger than the other. Sometimes the difference is very noticeable, as if one breast has hardly developed at all. From the breast-feeding point of view, this is not a problem – the small breast usually produces milk normally – but if you feel self-conscious about it, you could consider surgery. Usually the small breast is enlarged by an implant, and sometimes the size of the larger breast is reduced as well.

Small breasts

No exercise, electrical stimulation, creams or massage treatments will increase breast size. Women with large breasts often find that they become much larger with hormone treatments, such as the oral contraceptive pill or hormone replacement therapy, or during pregnancy. This does not usually happen if the breasts were small to start with.

Breast implant surgery (breast augmentation) is the only method of making breasts larger. It is obviously essential that the surgeon is reputable. Talk to your doctor about it. It is unlikely that your insurance will cover it – this is normally possible only if the breast is being reconstructed after breast cancer surgery, or if one breast is very under-developed compared with the other. Ask the surgeon to explain all the possible risks. If you do not understand the explanation, ask the surgeon to explain more clearly. After your discussion with the surgeon, go home and consider the information for a few days. (In fact the official recommendation is that there should be a 'cooling off' period of several days between seeing the surgeon and having the operation, to allow you to change your mind.)

- Breast enlargement is one of the most commonly performed cosmetic surgery operations.
- About 25,000 breast enlargement operations are done in the UK each year.
- In the US, there are about 2 million women whose breasts are not entirely their own, and about 150,000 in the UK.

The implant is placed behind the breast tissue, between it and the chest wall muscle (though very occasionally, it is placed behind the chest wall muscle, between the muscle and the ribcage). It is never placed in the breast tissue, so it does not interfere with the function of the breast and you can breast-feed later on if you wish. The implants come in a great variety of sizes, so it will be possible to use an implant which is the right size to make your breasts look similar.

There will be a skin scar in the crease line under the breast; this will be red at first

Breast implant in position

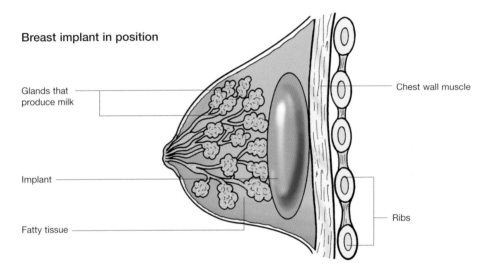

Glands that produce milk

Chest wall muscle

Implant

Ribs

Fatty tissue

but will gradually fade over 12 months. If a saline implant is used, some surgeons will be able to insert the bag of the implant by keyhole surgery (endoscopically) through an incision in the armpit. The bag is gradually filled with saline afterwards, and this technique means there is no scar on the actual breast.

Problems with breast enlargement surgery
- After the operation there will be some discomfort on moving the arms, but this wears off after a week or two.
- Occasionally blood collects round the implant in the first 24 hours after surgery, and the surgeon may have to re-open the incision to remove the blood.
- Infections can occur. Usually these can be dealt with by antibiotics, but if the

infection is severe the implant may need to be removed and replaced a couple of months later.

- The nipple may feel sore, or there may be loss of feeling in the nipple area. These are temporary phenomena.
- The scarred skin may become red and thick, and may stay like this for a year or two before starting to fade slowly.
- Tissue may tighten round the implant, squeezing it and making it feel much firmer. This used to be a common problem, but occurs less often with modern implants which have a textured surface. If it happens, you may need another operation.

Types of implant

Silicone-gel implants are still the most common, although they have had bad press in recent years. In particular, there has been much focus on leakage causing connective tissue diseases (arthritis-like diseases such as systemic lupus erythematosus or scleroderma). There is no clear evidence that this happens. A study published in the *British Medical Journal* in 1998, found no increase in connective tissue diseases in women with silicone implants. Leakage can, however, cause painful hardening of the breasts. In any case, these implants now have a stronger casing to reduce the risk of leakage.

Silicone-gel implants show up as a shadow on X-rays. This means a cancer cannot be detected easily by mammography in a person who has had an implant, and the breast has to be screened from special angles – if you have a mammogram, mention the implant to the radiologist.

Saline implants may be safer than silicone-gel, but they tend to leak (which will mean another operation) and may also produce a rippled effect under the skin. They cause the same difficulties with mammography as the silicone type.

Soya-oil implants have been used for only a few years, so not much is known about how well they last, or if they have any bad effects. Like the saline type, they can produce a rippled effect under the skin.

Tissue grown from our own bodies may be used as implants in the future. Researchers in the US have grown fatty tissue from laboratory rats in test tubes, and then implanted it successfully under the skin of the rats, where it developed its own blood supply.

Large breasts

Disproportionately large breasts can make a woman self-conscious. They can cause backache, probably because of adopting a drooping posture to try to hide their size. After a few years, the pressure from bra straps may cause grooves in the shoulders. High-impact sports such as jogging or aerobics can be uncomfortable or impossible. Clothes that fit properly can be hard to find. The oral contraceptive pill may have to be abandoned because it makes the breasts even larger.

The first essential is a well-fitting bra. Women with large breasts often make the mistake of choosing a large size with too small a cup, rather than a smaller size with a larger cup. For example, a woman who needs a 34E often buys a 36C.

Choosing a bra

- If the straps dig into your shoulders, the bra back size is probably too big, as the main support for the breasts should come from the strap around your body and the cups.
- If your bra rides up your back, the bra is too big around your body – the strap should fit around your ribcage.
- If your bra wrinkles, your cup size is too big – the breasts should be in the cups with a smooth outline.
- If your breasts bulge out of the top or sides of your cup, and your bra looks lumpy under clothes, your cup size is too small.
- If wires poke out at the front or dig in under your arms, the cup size is too small – the wires should lie flat against your body and surround your breasts.

Discuss the pros and cons of breast reduction surgery with your doctor. This does not commit you to anything, and may help you decide whether you can come to terms with your figure – and see it as an advantage – or whether you would really like surgery. It is unlikely that you would be able to have your insurance pay for the operation.

Breast reduction surgery is a more complicated operation than breast enlargement with implants, and takes 2 or 3 hours. Skill is needed to make both breasts look the same shape. The operation is more 'final' as it cannot be reversed. It is not surprising that far fewer breast reduction operations than breast enlarging operations are performed.

As with breast enlargement surgery, it is important to find a skilled surgeon. Within reason, the surgeon can remove as much or as little as you want, so you should end up with breasts the size you like.

The surgeon removes a wedge of breast tissue and reshapes the remaining skin and tissue. The nipple will have to be moved to a new position. Therefore there will be scars right round the nipple, in the crease line under the breast and along a line joining the nipple to the crease line. These scars take about a year to fade. The scar around the nipple fades first.

Problems with breast reduction surgery

- There is often some loss of feeling from the nipple – often touch can be felt, but there may be loss of erotic feeling.
- Breast-feeding may not be possible afterwards.
- The incisions may take a long time to heal, especially round the nipple, and the central part of the incision in the crease line.
- The scars from the incisions usually fade in 6–12 months but can become thickened and unsightly.

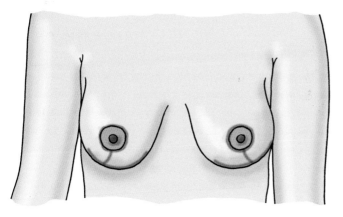

Scars after breast reduction surgery or mastoplexy

Drooping breasts

It is natural for breasts to droop with age, especially in women with large breasts who have had several pregnancies.

Treatments that don't work

Breasts do not contain any muscle within them, so no exercises will improve matters. Cosmetic companies and private clinics have realized that huge numbers of women are self-conscious about drooping breasts, and offer dubious and expensive 'treatments'. For example, some clinics offer 'non-surgical breast lifts' using electrical (*galvanic*) stimulation to 'tone and lift the breasts'; this cannot and does not work. Many 'firming' gels and lotions are available; these simply tighten the skin and so give a temporary sensation of breast firmness. Some claim that they contain elastin or collagen, the body's structural proteins; in fact, elastin or collagen applied to the surface of the skin will not be absorbed through it.

Surgery. Very drooping breasts can be tightened up by surgery. This is called *mastoplexy*. The surgeon removes a wedge of skin and tissue from the loose, saggy upper part of the breasts. The nipple and the breast tissue underneath it has to be moved so that the nipple is positioned in the skin further up than it was. There will be a scar around the nipple area, a scar running from the nipple to the crease line underneath the breast, and sometimes a small scar in the crease line (see preceding page). The breasts end up the same size as before, but have a more pleasing shape.

As with all cosmetic breast surgery, it is important to choose a reputable surgeon (see page 45).

Redness under the breasts

A red 'sweat rash' under the breasts is called *intertrigo*. It may be sore and itchy, and you may have it in the armpits as well. The rash has a definite edge, and there may be some whitish material on it. It is usually caused by *Candida* fungus, which likes to live in warm, moist places. If you are overweight as well as having large breasts, the skin crease underneath them is ideal for *Candida*. *Candida* also likes skin that has been slightly damaged; this makes it easier for the fungus to take hold.

To improve the situation, get a supportive bra to lift your breasts up, preferably made from cotton to absorb sweat. Wash carefully with a non-perfumed soap (some perfumes can damage the skin). Don't put any disinfectants in the water. Rinse well to ensure no lather remains in the skin crease. Dry thoroughly but gently – pat dry with a soft towel or use a hairdryer. Don't wash your hair with shampoo in the shower – the shampoo may trickle down to under your breasts, and may contain irritant perfume.

If you have been applying creams from the pharmacist, stop using them, even if they say 'for *Candida*' on the label. You could have become sensitized to one of the ingredients, and the cream could be making it worse. Instead, simply follow the instructions above for 2 weeks. If at the end of that time the rash is no better, see your doctor who will be able to prescribe a different cream. You may find the rash difficult to eliminate completely unless you lose some weight.

Painful breasts

Nearly all women have tender, painful breasts at some time during their life. If you suffer from regular pain, ask yourself these two important questions:

- is the pain related to the menstrual cycle (is it worse before your period?)
- are both breasts affected, or just one?

You can check these points by keeping a daily diary over 2 or 3 months. Every day, record whether or not you have any breast pain, whether it is mild or severe and which breast is affected. Also make a note of the days of your period.

Breast pain related to the menstrual cycle (*cyclical breast pain*)

It is common to have painful, heavy, bloated breasts before a period. Both breasts are affected at the same time. The breasts may feel generally lumpy but there isn't one particular lump. If you are particularly unlucky, it may be so bad you cannot bear to be touched, are pain-free for only a few days each month, or have to wear a bra at night because it is so tender when you lie on your side in bed.

Causes. Cyclical breast pain affecting both breasts is not a symptom of breast cancer. It occurs because some women's breasts are particularly sensitive to hormone changes. Each breast is made up of a collection of glands for producing milk; these are rather like

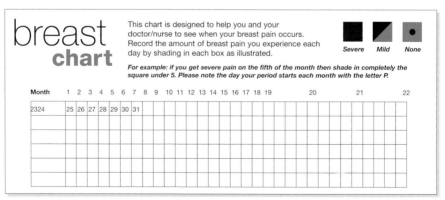

Reproduced with kind permission of Professor R E Mansel, University of Wales College of Medicine.

bunches of silky white grapes. The 'stalks' of the bunches are small milk ducts, which lead into larger and larger ducts for the milk to reach the surface of the nipple. The glands are supported and padded in 'packing tissue', which is mostly fat. Each month the glands respond to the rise and fall of hormones. It used to be thought that the problem was caused by fluid retained in the packing tissue, but this has been disproved.

What you can do:
- Wear a soft bra at night
- Avoid jogging, aerobics or other high-impact exercises
- Make sure your bra fits correctly (see page 48) – get properly measured by a specialist fitter; most department stores have one
- If you are taking any hormones – the oral contraceptive pill, or hormone replacement therapy – consider stopping them for a while to see if the breast pain lessens.

There is some evidence that high levels of saturated fats in the blood make the breasts more sensitive to hormone levels, so it may be worth changing your diet. Avoid fatty meat, cheese, full-fat milk, cream, butter and anything made of pastry. Instead eat oily fish, such as herring and mackerel, twice a week. Fill up with carbohydrates (bread, potatoes, rice, pasta), fresh fruit and vegetables. It has also been suggested that caffeine worsens breast pain, so try avoiding coffee and cola drinks for a few weeks to see if it makes any difference.

What your doctor can do. Most of the treatments for cyclical breast pain take several months to work, so you have to be patient. Continue your diary while starting any treatment; this will help you to decide whether it is having any effect. If any treatment works, it is usually continued for about 6 months and then stopped. In 50% of women, the pain will not recur; if it does, further treatment can be given.

Your doctor can prescribe gamma linolenic acid, the active ingredient of evening primrose oil. Three to four capsules are usually taken twice a day for 8–12 weeks; it may take this long to have any effect and the improvement is usually gradual. If it works, the dose is then reduced. It can sometimes cause nausea and indigestion, but has no other side-effects. Of women who take this treatment, 30–40% find their condition improves.

The next step is hormone treatment such as bromocriptine or danazol. Bromocriptine reduces the level of the hormone prolactin, which stimulates breast tissue to grow. Bromocriptine works in about half of women, but a third of people taking it develop side-effects such as nausea, headache, constipation, and dizziness when they stand up suddenly.

The drug danazol has several different effects on the hormone system. In the breast it may block the effects of hormones such as progesterone. It works in about 70% of women with breast pain, and works more quickly than the other treatments. It has some side-effects such as irregular periods, weight gain, headache, nausea, acne, oily skin and sometimes deepening of the voice. These effects can be minimized by taking it only for the 7 days before a period.

Clinic treatments. If no treatments seem to help after 4 months, ask for a referral to a specialist breast clinic. Some clinics prescribe drugs related to testosterone (the male hormone), such as Restandol. These can have some masculinizing side-effects and would usually be prescribed for only a short period (for example, 3 months).

Tamoxifen is another possibility. This drug counteracts estrogen and is often used for breast cancer, but sometimes a low dose is used for breast pain not caused by cancer (although it is not officially licensed for this purpose at the moment) – so if the specialist suggests that you take tamoxifen, do not assume that you have cancer. It must not be taken during pregnancy, so effective contraception is essential.

Recently, massaging the breasts with ibuprofen gel has been reported to produce dramatic improvements. This is a non-steroidal anti-inflammatory gel, and is usually used for sprains and rheumatic pains. Researchers are not sure whether it is the drug itself that produces the benefit, or whether it is simply the effect of the massage.

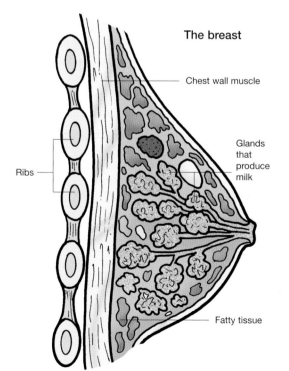

The breast

Chest wall muscle

Glands that produce milk

Ribs

Fatty tissue

Treatments that don't really work

- Diuretics don't work, because the pain is not caused by fluid retention.
- Vitamin B_6 is sometimes prescribed if gamma linolenic acid does not help, before moving on to hormone treatment. However, studies have shown that although about 30% of women find that it helps, the same number reported improvement with a placebo (dummy tablet), so its effect is probably psychological. High intakes of vitamin B_6 of more than 10 mg/day over a long period may cause nerve damage.
- Antibiotics are pointless; there is no infection
- Progesterone hormone has been tried in tablet form and as a breast cream, but there is no evidence it does any good (apart from having a psychological effect).

Pain unrelated to the menstrual cycle (*non-cyclical breast pain*)

If your breast pain has no monthly pattern and occurs in just one breast, it is known as non-cyclical breast pain and shouldn't be ignored. Rather than a heavy, bloated, tender feeling, this type of pain tends to be sharp or burning. There is usually a very simple cause such as bruising from an injury, a sports strain, an infection such as shingles or a breast abcess, a viral infection of the muscles between the ribs (Bornholm disease), inflammation of the joint between the front of a rib and the breastbone (Tietze's syndrome), a lung problem such as pleurisy, or even gallstones. However, there is a very faint chance that it could be related to early breast cancer, so you should check it out with your doctor.

Breasts in men

The breasts can enlarge if you are overweight, simply because fat has settled there. They can also enlarge because of overdevelopment of the actual breast tissue; this is called *gynaecomastia.*

To decide which it is, lie flat and grasp your 'breast' tightly between your thumb and forefinger. Then gradually move your finger and thumb towards the nipple. If you can feel a firm, rubbery disk-like mound of tissue which is more than 2 cm across, and which seems to be stuck to the back of the nipple and to the pink area surrounding the nipple *(areola),* it is likely that the breast tissue is overdeveloped. The area may feel tender. Usually both breasts are equally affected, but sometimes development of one is more obvious than the other. If there is no distinct mound of tissue under the nipple, it may simply be that you are too fat.

How breasts develop

Even a newborn baby has some basic breast tissue, which started to develop when it was a 6-week-old fetus. Before puberty, the breasts are the same in girls and boys. They consist of tiny branching tubes embedded in packing tissue. The glands (see page 53) for making milk have not yet formed.

At puberty, hormone levels start to rise. In females, the main hormone is estrogen (the 'female hormone'). Estrogen makes the tubes thicken, lengthen and become more branched, and also stimulates the development of glandular lobules.

In men, the main sexual hormone is testosterone. This is made mainly in the testicles. The level of testosterone rises at puberty to 30 times the level it was before. Men normally also have a small amount of estrogen; at puberty it rises to only three times the level it was before. This estrogen often makes the breast tissue grow slightly in teenage boys (see below), but eventually the high levels of testosterone take over completely and prevent the estrogen having any further effect on the breast. Therefore glandular lobules do not form in men. Instead, the breasts flatten out, and remain as a collection of tubes in packing tissue, just as they were before puberty.

Breast growth in teenage boys

Teenage boys sometimes notice that their breasts are enlarging and/or are tender. This is nothing to worry about, and happens to about half of all boys at some time (see below). It does not mean you are changing sex! It can start anytime after the age of about 10, and the breasts may be quite large by age 13–14. In the mid-to-late teens, they start to become smaller again, and will usually have flattened out by age 18 or 19.

Results of some surveys of breast enlargement in normal teenage boys	
Normal teenage boys examined	Those with breast enlargement
1865 American scouts, aged 10–16	39%
993 Turkish schoolboys, aged 9–17	7%
29 American schoolboys, at puberty	69%
681 Italian schoolboys, aged 11–14	33%
135 Swiss youths, aged $8^1/_2$–$17^1/_2$	22%
377 American schoolboys, aged 10–15	49%

(Source: *New England Journal of Medicine* 1993;328:490–5)

Why it happens. At puberty, the testosterone level does not rise steadily. Over the first few teenage years it fluctuates wildly all the time, and on some days the level will dip quite low. These dips in testosterone allow the small amount of estrogen, which is circulating in the blood of all men, to have an effect on the breast. This estrogen stimulates the growth of the packing tissue and tubes, so that the breasts enlarge. Above about 15 years of age, the testosterone settles at a more steady, high level. This prevents the estrogen from having any more effect, and the breast tissue starts to shrink.

What if the breasts remain enlarged? In just a few men the breasts remain enlarged at the end of the teen years. This is rarely because there is anything wrong with the male hormones. It usually means that for some reason the enlarged breast tissue is still hypersensitive to the tiny normal amounts of oestrogen, or else is not responsive to the 'shutting down' effect of testosterone. Your doctor can check your hormone levels, and if everything is normal (which it usually is) the excess breast tissue can be removed by a surgeon.

Causes of breast enlargement in men
It seems that breast tissue is very sensitive to the balance between estrogen and testosterone in the blood. If there is either a fall in the testosterone level or a rise in the estrogen level, the breasts will be stimulated to grow.

Obesity is a common cause. If you are overweight, the breasts will of course be larger because they are more fatty. In addition, fat produces oestrogen which stimulates breast development.

Drugs are the other most likely reason. Some drugs have an estrogen-like effect on the breast, and some block the effect of testosterone. Estrogens are easily absorbed through the skin; men have developed breasts after using anti-balding scalp creams containing estrogen, and even by absorption through the skin of the penis from a partner using a vaginal oestrogen cream.

Alcohol abuse upsets both sides of the estrogen:testosterone balance. It stimulates the liver to clear testosterone out of the blood, so testosterone levels fall. It probably also reduces the ability of the liver to break down estrogens, so estrogen levels rise. Fortunately the liver can often recover if alcohol intake is reduced.

Tumors are rare causes of breast enlargement. Breast cancer can occur in the male breast, but is usually on only one side. Tumors in other parts of the body can sometimes produce hormones that make the breasts grow and may also cause impotence and/or oozing of milk from the breast; if you have these symptoms it is vital to see your doctor right away.

Old age. It is natural for men's breasts to enlarge in old age. This is partly because less testosterone is produced. Also, in old age the body often contains a higher proportion of fat, which produces estrogens.

Drugs that can cause breast enlargement in men	
Hormones	Estrogen
	Anabolic (body-building) steroids
Drugs for hypertension or heart problems	Calcium channel blockers (for example, nifedipine)
	ACE inhibitors (for example, captopril, enalapril)
	Digoxin
	Amiodarone
	Spironolactone
	Methyldopa
Psychiatric drugs	Phenothiazines (for example, chlorpromazine)
	Tricyclic antidepressants (for example, amitriptyline)
	Benzodiazepines (for example, diazepam)
	Opiates
Drug misuse	Alcohol
	Marijuana
	Heroin
	Amphetamines
Antibiotics and antifungal drugs	Isoniazid
	Metronidazole
	Ketoconazole
Drugs for duodenal ulcer	Omeprazole
	Cimetidine
Some anti-cancer drugs	

What your doctor can do

See your doctor if you think your breasts are enlarging, even if you have worked out the most likely cause. Your doctor will be able to:

- Check whether the actual glandular breast tissue is overdeveloped, or whether the enlargement is simply fat
- Check your testicles (because they make most of the testosterone)
- Decide whether any drugs are likely to be responsible
- Do blood tests to measure various hormones, including testosterone.

The treatment will depend on the reason. It may simply be a matter of losing weight or cutting down your alcohol intake. If the problem is a low testosterone level, testosterone can be given by injection or as a patch. Tamoxifen – a drug that interferes with the action of estrogen – is used by some specialists to reduce gynaecomastia. Another possibility is danazol, a drug that promotes the effect of testosterone. Danazol can have troublesome side-effects, such as weight gain, acne, muscle cramps and nausea. The excess breast tissue can also be removed by surgery.

USEFUL CONTACTS

The American Cancer Society offers many resources for women with breast cancer, including links to support groups, breast cancer websites, fact sheets, and publications about breast cancer.
Call toll-free:
1-800-ACS-2345
www.cancer.org

WIN Against Breast Cancer (Women's Information Network)
536 S. Second Avenue, Suite K
Covina, California 91723-3043
By Phone: (626) 332-2255
By Fax: (626) 332-2585
www.winabc.org

The Susan G. Komen Breast Cancer Foundation
5005 LBJ Freeway
Suite 250
Dallas, TX   75244
Phone: 972.855.1600
FAX: 972.855.1605
www.komen.org

condoms

"I hate using condoms, because I wilt while I'm trying to put it on"

- Early condoms were made of linen or pig or sheep's gut, tied at the end with ribbon. After sex, they were rinsed out and reused!
- An 18th-century illustrated condom, featuring three naughty nuns, was sold at a Christie's auction for $5000
- There is no truth in the story that condoms were invented by a Dr. Condom, physician to Charles II
- Although it has been suggested that condoms were used by the Ancient Egyptians, the earliest actual report of a condom was by the Italian anatomist, Fallapio in 1564. He claimed to have invented a linen sheath, made to fit the penis, as protection against syphilis
- In England, condoms are known as 'French Letters'. In Italy they used to be called 'English Overcoats'

Problems putting it on

Condom manufacturers never mention this problem in their brochures. They simply tell you to unroll it onto the hard and erect penis, and preferably to pinch the closed end to keep it empty at the same time. To do this properly you need three hands or the assistance of a cooperative partner. It is no wonder that a survey conducted by the University of Sydney, Australia – which asked men about what *really* happened when they used condoms – found that two-thirds of them sometimes or often lost their erection while trying to put the condom on, so it was then impossible to put it on properly. Many disliked using a condom because it drew attention to this wilting problem.

The researchers suggest that, to make things easier for yourself, you should not try to pinch the end of the condom as you put it on. They found that pinching the end makes no difference to the likelihood of the condom breaking or slipping off during intercourse. Latex condoms are designed to stretch enormously, so there is no reason why the presence of 1 ml or so of air in addition to 3–5 ml of semen should 'burst' the condom. They also suggest

Wise-up to condoms

Do:

- buy your condoms from a pharmacist or reputable brand vending machine or other reliable source, not from a street trader
- check the sell-by date when you buy – the further ahead it is, the better
- choose a reputable brand that has an expiration date of over 2 years. Expiration dates are usually 5 years after manufacture.
- make sure you have several with you, in case you damage one or it goes on wrongly
- be careful as you unwrap the condom – they can be damaged by teeth, fingernails or jewelry
- use a water-based lubricant if needed, such as KY Jelly
- put the condom on before your penis touches your partner's genitals. It is possible for a woman to become pregnant if any sperm are spilled near the entrance of the vagina even if you do not have full intercourse. Sperm can ooze out of the penis before ejaculation happens
- remember that the more you use condoms, and the more familiar you are with them, the more comfortable and efficient you will become

Don't:

- use a condom that is past its sell-by date or which feels sticky or very dry
- rely on a gimmick condom (glow-in the-dark, musical etc.) for contraception
- use Vaseline, handcream, butter, baby oil or any other oils for lubrication; oil can cause the rubber to break down, and can reduce the strength of the condom by up to 95% in 15 minutes. (Some condoms are made from polyurethane; these are resistant to oils)
- use a condom more than once; use a new one each time you have intercourse

that instead of rolling the condom on, as suggested by the manufacturers, you could try pulling it on like a sock with your thumbs or fingers inside. Using this method, you can put it on securely even if your penis is not fully rigid. Obviously you have to be careful not to damage it with your nails. In their study, the researchers found that people who used this method had less chance of the condom slipping off or breaking.

Slipping off

If you find a condom slips off, you probably assume it is too large for you. In fact, it is probably too small. If the condom is too tight you probably aren't unrolling it fully down the penis. This means that, during intercourse, the ring at the base of the condom is entering your partner's vagina, where it can be dragged off. If the condom is the right size, the ring will be right at the base of your penis, and will remain outside the vagina during sex.

If you have difficulty putting the condom on properly try the 'pull-on' method (see preceding page). Finding the right size may be a matter of trial and error, because only a few manufacturers clearly show the length and width on the pack. The other problem is that most men don't really know how the size of their erect penis compares with other men, so don't know whether they need a large condom or not. And most men only consider length whereas, just like short fat legs in stockings, a short fat penis needs a large condom.

After ejaculation, when the penis quickly becomes limp, the condom can easily slip off, spilling sperm into your partner's vagina. At this stage you must hold the condom firmly around the penis so that it remains in place until you have withdrawn.

Breaking

The University of Sydney, Australia, ran a study of condom breakage in three brothels. They supplied the fresh condoms, together with forms to fill in if there was an accident and little plastic bags to put the torn condoms in so the researchers could analyze in the laboratory how and why they tore. Of the 1269 condoms the workers used, only eight were reported broken and two of these turned out to be intact when they were examined. Next, they did a survey of ordinary men, and found that their breakage rates were far higher than for the sex workers – about 7% (although this included breakages while putting the condoms on). They found that men were likely to break more condoms if they didn't use condoms often, and if they rolled the condom on rather than pulled it on (see preceding pages).

Another reason for breakage may be lack of lubrication. Condom manufacturers admit that the lubrication that they put on their condoms may not be enough, but adding more would make packaging difficult. Prostitutes tend to use additional lubrication, which may be another reason for their lower breakage rate.

Most condoms are made from latex (rubber). With these, choose a water-based, oil-free lubricant (such as KY Jelly), because oil dissolves rubber and makes breakage more likely. For the same reason, don't let massage oil or handcreams come into contact with the condom. Some medication creams for vaginal or rectal problems can also weaken latex condoms. Condoms made from polyurethane (which is different from latex) are available (check the packet). These are not damaged by oily substances.

Emergency contraception – used to be called the *morning-after* pill

- Emergency contraception prevents pregnancy after intercourse has occurred – so it is a back-up if another method fails (such as when a condom breaks or slips off, or you forget a pill).

- In fact it can be taken up to 72 hours after intercourse – not just on the morning after.

- The main side-effect is nausea (in 50%) and vomiting (in 20%).

- It usually consists of two doses, taken 12 hours apart.

- You can obtain it from your doctor or from a family planning clinic.

- The next period is unpredictable – it might be earlier or later than usual. Emergency contraception doesn't always work, so if your next period is late you might be pregnant – have a pregnancy test to check.

What to do if a condom slips or breaks

If a condom slips off during intercourse, or if it breaks, the woman should visit her doctor or a family planning clinic as soon as possible for emergency contraception.

USEFUL CONTACTS

Planned Parenthood Federation of America offers information about contraception, including the "morning-after" pill.

810 Seventh Ave.
New York, NY 10019
212/541-7800
FAX. 212/246-1845
communications@ppfa.org
www.plannedparenthood.org

Family planning clinics – look in the telephone directory under 'Family Planning' for your local clinic.

crab lice

- The French used to call crab lice 'papillons d'amour', which means 'butterflies of love'
- Lice have been found on 4000-year-old mummies
- Lousy, nitwit, nit-picking, nitty-gritty, go through something with a fine tooth-comb – all these phrases come from lice
- In medieval Gothenburg, in Sweden, lice helped to choose the mayor. Candidates sat round the table with their beards on the table. A louse was put in the centre and the owner of the beard it crawled into became the new mayor – a virile man was supposed to attract lice!

Lice feed on human blood. There are three types – head lice (common in children), body lice (common in vagrants, live in clothing and only visit the skin to feed), and pubic (crab) lice.

Ways of knowing you have crab lice
- Itching – especially at night, in the pubic hair area.
- Seeing the lice – they are tiny, but can just be seen with the naked eye. They are squat in shape, and with a magnifier you can see that all the legs emerge close together from the front of the body, and the middle and hind legs have large pincer-like claws – giving the 'crab' appearance. They use their claws to grasp hairs close to the skin surface. They hardly move except at night, when they slowly transfer their grip from one hair to another.
- Nits – these are egg-cases, attached to the hairs. The female lays the eggs in a hard brown shell, which she attaches to the hair on the surface of the skin. As the hair grows, the egg case will be further up its shaft, so the position of the nits on the hair gives you an idea of how long you have had them. After about 8 days the eggs hatch, and the empty egg case appears white and is easier to see.
- Rust-colored specks on the skin – these are louse feces.
- Blood specks on underwear.

How lice are caught

Lice cannot jump, hop, fly or swim. Crab lice are relatively helpless when removed from the skin, and a crab louse that has lost its grip usually does so permanently. This means that crab lice probably cannot be caught from lavatory seats or even from bedclothes. They are transmitted by close body contact, during which they are able to transfer their grip from one person's hair to that of the other before letting go entirely from the first person. Sexual contact is their ideal situation.

Crab lice cannot survive in hair that is too dense, so they will not colonize the hair of the scalp (except at the hairline). However, they will live happily on armpit hair, eyebrows, eyelashes, chest hair and upper thigh hair as well as pubic hair.

Treatment

For treatment, you have a choice. You can buy a standard treatment without a prescription from the pharmacy. Most of these treatments contain alcohol, which can irritate the skin of the scrotum and any scratched areas.

Alternatively you can see your doctor or go to a health clinic. The advantage of the clinic is that the staff are expert crab spotters who will be able to confirm that your diagnosis is correct. Also, you can have tests to check you haven't picked up any other infection at the same time, and the treatment will probably be free. Definitely go to a clinic if you think you have crabs on your eyelashes or eyebrows: don't try to treat these yourself with lotion.

A single application of a prescription lotion is probably enough, but some specialists advise another application after 7 days to eliminate any newly hatched lice. Apply the lotion to the *whole body* from the neck down, even if you think only the pubic area is affected. A paintbrush is the best method. To be on the safe side, change underclothes and bed linen after treatment.

dandruff

Dandruff particles are visible flakes of skin that have been continuously shed from the scalp. It is normal to shed some dead skin flakes as the skin is constantly renewing itself. The new cells form in the lower layers and are gradually pushed to the surface as more new cells form beneath them. By the time they reach the surface the cells have become flat, and overlap each other like plates. These cells are in fact dead, and are shed from the surface all the time. They are so small that we do not notice them. With dandruff, this whole process of renewal (*skin turnover*) speeds up, so a greater number of dead cells are being shed. Also, the cells are shed in clumps, which are big enough to be seen with the naked eye as embarrassing flakes, especially when they land on dark clothing. The scalp may feel slightly itchy.

The cause of dandruff

Surprisingly, dandruff is a bit of an enigma. About 10 years ago, dermatologists discovered that people with dandruff have large numbers of a tiny yeast, *Pityrosporum ovale*, on the scalp. Everyone has some of this yeast on their skin – particularly in the greasy areas such as the scalp and upper back – but people with dandruff have a lot of it. However, it is not known which comes first – whether the yeast actually causes the increased turnover and flaking, or whether the flaky skin simply provides an ideal environment for the yeast to thrive. It seems very likely that the former is the case, so getting rid of the yeast should improve the dandruff.

Getting rid of dandruff

- If your dandruff is mild, try shampooing your hair twice a week using any shampoo labelled 'frequent use, for dry hair' (not an 'anti-dandruff' shampoo). This will remove the flakes that are being shed, and the moisturizer in the shampoo will protect the scalp.
- For more severe dandruff, you need to deal with the yeast. Look for a shampoo (for example, Head 'n Shoulders, Selsun Blue) containing selenium sulphide, which has an anti-yeast effect and is available without a prescription. Don't use selenium sulphide within 48 hours of applying a hair dye or a perm lotion.

- The most effective treatment is an anti-yeast shampoo containing ketoconazole, but you need a doctor's prescription for this. You should certainly see your doctor if your scalp is red and itchy – or if the skin is flaky around the eyebrows, round the nose or behind the ears – because this suggests you have the more severe form called *seborrhoeic dermatitis.*

ears that stick out

"My ears stick out – am I too old for an operation?"

Ears are one of the first parts of the body to reach full size – by the age of 5 or 6 our ears are about the size they will be when we are adults. This is why ears that stick out are particularly noticeable in children, and an operation (called *otoplasty*) to correct the problem is often done when the child is over 5 or 6. However, there is no reason why it cannot be done at any age.

What is involved

Children need a general anesthetic, but adults can have the operation with just a local anesthetic. The surgeon cuts away skin and tissue from behind each ear, and stitches it into its new position. The ears are bandaged for about 10 days after the operation, and after that the stitches are removed. You will have to wear a headband at night for the next 2 weeks so that you do not accidentally bend the ears forward during sleep.

As with any cosmetic surgery operation, it is important to find a plastic surgeon who is skilled at this particular operation (For advice on plastic surgeons, see page 45). If it is clumsily done, you may end up with a 'plastered-down' look, or with ears that don't look the same.

ejaculation

- Each milliliter of semen normally contains at least 20 million sperm and can contain up to 100 million
- The average ejaculation is about 5 ml (a teaspoonful) and contains about 300 million sperm
- Semen is made up of 5% sperm from the testicles, 35% fluid from the prostate gland and 60% fluid from the seminal vesicle glands

Not enough semen

The sensation of orgasm is a relief of tension beginning just before the semen starts to spurt out, and ending with the final spurt – so if there is not much semen the orgasm will be short. Most men ejaculate more fluid at some times than at others – the amount can vary from a few drops to two teaspoonfuls. Some medical conditions can produce *dry orgasm*. For example, this can occur after surgery to the prostate gland, or with diabetes or some drugs. If your dry orgasm is due to prostate surgery, the volume cannot be increased.

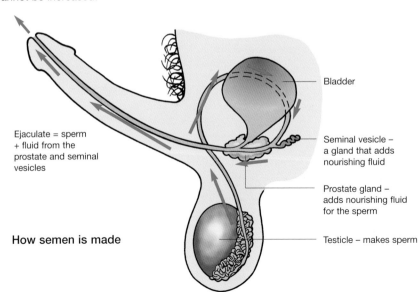

Ejaculate = sperm + fluid from the prostate and seminal vesicles

Bladder

Seminal vesicle – a gland that adds nourishing fluid

Prostate gland – adds nourishing fluid for the sperm

How semen is made

Testicle – makes sperm

What to do:

- Abstain from sex for a few days. Unless it is due to a medical condition, the volume of ejaculate can be increased in this way.
- Try to delay ejaculation for as long as possible during intercourse. Much of the fluid is produced during the state of arousal before ejaculation.
- If you think that a drug you are taking is responsible, ask your doctor if an alternative drug is available.

Premature ejaculation

Ejaculation is the peak of male orgasm, when the semen is released. For years, sex therapists have been arguing about the precise definition of 'premature' ejaculation. In the 1950s, a man was said to be a premature ejaculator if he lasted less than a certain time (say 2 minutes) or a certain number of strokes (say 100) before ejaculating. These arbitrary definitions are rubbish; they were based on ignorance of how long most men actually take to climax. The so-called 'experts' were surprised when Dr Alfred Kinsey reported that 75% of men ejaculate within 2 minutes of vaginal penetration. Similarly, in Shere Hite's survey of 11,239 men, 21% reported that they ejaculated within 1 minute of penetration, and 62% within 5 minutes. The Hite survey also showed that there is great variation between men: for example, 7% said they did not ejaculate before 15 minutes.

The best definition of premature ejaculation is climaxing before you or your partner wish you to. This common-sense definition means that climaxing speedily after penetration is not necessarily a problem (for example, if a man pleasures his partner for a long time beforehand until she reaches orgasm). On the other hand, many men and their partners wish to last longer than they do. In the Hite survey, about 70% of men said 'yes' to the question 'Do you ever orgasm too soon after penetration – in other words, are you unable to continue intercourse for as long as you would like?'

What causes it?

It used to be thought that premature ejaculation was the result of a physical problem such as irritation or inflammation of the urethra (the tube in the penis for urine and semen) or prostate gland, and there were nasty treatments such as squirting silver nitrate into the opening. There is no evidence that premature ejaculation is caused by such conditions. Very rarely, it can be the result of neurological conditions such as multiple sclerosis.

Common-sense measures for premature ejaculation

- Have sex more often – you are more likely to ejaculate prematurely after a long gap.
- For the same reason, masturbating before intercourse may help.
- Use a condom to decrease sensation.
- Have sex with the woman on top – men are less aroused in this position than when they are on top ('missionary position').
- Learn to control your anal muscles. Contract your buttocks around the anus as if you were trying to prevent a bowel movement. Start by doing this 10 times in a row, and increase to 50 times twice a day. Some men find either contracting or relaxing these muscles when ejaculation is near helps them to last longer.
- When your penis is first inside your partner's vagina, try to make shorter thrusts or a circular motion – this can delay ejaculation and you can then progress to the usual in-and-out technique when you and your partner are ready.

There is also no evidence that it happens because the penis is hypersensitive. Researchers tested the sensitivity of the skin of the penis in men who considered themselves premature ejaculators and men who were not, and found no difference. It also seems to be a myth that circumcision makes a difference; the American sex researchers Masters and Johnson tested the sensitivity of the glans (head) of the penis in circumcised and non-circumcised men and found them to be the same. It is most likely that the time of ejaculation is simply a habit, starting early when a youth learns to masturbate or have sex as quickly as possible for fear of being caught. Like all habits, it can be unlearned. Common-sense measures may help.

'Unlearning' premature ejaculation

The main methods are the so-called *squeeze technique* and *stop–go technique*. They involve stimulating the penis almost to the point of ejaculation and then stopping. The idea is to train the man to remain in a state of high arousal without actually ejaculating. They require patience. About 90% of men are 'cured' by these techniques but it usually takes about 14 weeks with practicing 3–5 times a week. Unfortunately about 60% find that the problem comes back after about a year, and the 'unlearning' has to be gone through again.

These techniques are not as easy as they sound, but do not despair. The usual problems are that the man goes too far and ejaculates, or he loses his erection and cannot regain it. If these occur, don't worry – just try again another day. It may take several weeks to master the techniques.

The next step is to do exactly the same, but using a lubricant jelly (such as KY jelly) to increase sensation and more closely resemble the situation of being in the vagina.

When you find that you are beginning to be able to delay ejaculation, you can start to have intercourse with the woman on top. She lowers herself backwards and downwards onto the erect penis and makes gentle coital movements. You signal to her when ejaculation is about to happen. She then remains perfectly still, or lifts herself off and either does nothing or applies the squeeze, before resuming intercourse in the same position.

Squeeze technique

- This is best done by the couple, but the man can do it alone by masturbation if there is no partner or she is not willing to participate.
- The couple start by being as relaxed as they can, and free from distractions.
- The couple kiss and caress until the man is aroused, and then she takes his penis in her hand and begins stroking it.
- The man concentrates on his feelings of arousal, to increase his sexual awareness. (He does not try to think of other things in an attempt to distract himself from ejaculation).
- When he feels he is about to ejaculate, he signals to his partner.
- She immediately stops stimulating him and applies firm but gentle pressure around the penis where the glans (head) meets the shaft. She applies this pressure for 10–20 seconds.
- She then lets go, and they wait without doing anything for about 30 seconds.
- The procedure is repeated several times before ejaculation is allowed to occur.

Stop–go technique

- This is essentially the same as the squeeze technique, but the squeeze is omitted.
- As soon as the man is about to ejaculate, he signals to his partner and she stops stroking his penis.
- It is simpler than the squeeze technique, and seems to work just as well.

Drugs

Antidepressants: clomipramine (Anafranil), fluoxetine (Prozac), sertraline (Lustral), and paroxetine (Seroxat) delay ejaculation as a side-effect, and some doctors prescribe them for this purpose.

Stud 100 is a local anesthetic spray which has been approved by the drug regulatory authorities in the US and UK. It is sprayed onto the *glans* (head) and shaft of the penis up to 10 minutes before intercourse. It is not very effective on its own, but is useful if you have successfully 'retrained' with the squeeze or stop–go techniques but feel that you are in danger of slipping back. A problem is that some of the local anesthetic may rub off onto the female partner, causing her genital area to lose some feeling temporarily.

USEFUL CONTACTS

Sexual Function Health Council
o/o American Foundation for Urologic Disease, Inc
1128 North Charles Street
Baltimore, MD 21201
(800) 433-4215
www.afud.org
www.impotence.org

National Kidney and Urologic Diseases Information Clearinghouse
3 Information Way
Bethesda, MD 20892-3580
(301) 654-4415
www.niddk.nih.gov

American Diabetes Association National Center
1660 Duke Street
Alexandria, VA 22314
(800) 232-3472
www.diabetes.org

Man-To-Man
American Cancer Society
1599 Clifton Road, N.E.
Atlanta, GA 30329
(800) 227-2345

fecal incontinence

*"I leave brown 'skid marks' on my underwear
– then I have to hide it in the laundry basket"*

The fact that 6.5% of normal people soil their underwear doesn't make it any
more pleasant.

Your diet

This is the first thing to check. Anything that makes the consistency of the feces more
runny – such as a heavy intake of beer – will make it more difficult for you to hold them
in. In the US, the 'non-fat fat', called Olestra, used in some 'slimming' foods has
gained unwelcome publicity for this reason. Olestra reportedly cost $200 million to
develop, and over $10 million in advertising and promotion. It is an artificial mixture of
fats, none of which can be digested or absorbed. Instead, it goes straight along the gut
and is passed out at the other end. This means that the feces are runny and slippery
with fat, and soiled underwear can result. Frito-Lay, the first company to market
Olestra-containing chips in the US, admits that Olestra caused 'anal oil leakage' in a
study commissioned by the company.

A new type of diet pill, called orlistat, works by blocking the enzymes that digest fat.
This means that the fat cannot be absorbed from the gut. With the correct dose, a third
of the fat that you eat is blocked, and is excreted in the feces instead of ending up as
part of your spare tire. But, as with Olestra, this extra fat in the gut can cause anal
leakage, and the problem gets worse the more fat you eat. Anything which makes you
pass more wind (see page 196) makes leakage more likely. This is because the anus
has to relax to let the wind out, and some fecal material may be propelled out at the
same time.

Irritable bowel syndrome

This is the other common cause. It is also known as IBS. If you have abdominal pain as well as leakage of feces, then this is a strong possibility. The pain of IBS can occur anywhere in the abdomen, but is usually felt low down on the right or left side. Passing wind or opening the bowels often relieves it. People with IBS often have to rush to the lavatory, and some leakage is common. There is also often a 'morning rush' – the bowels have to be opened urgently several times on rising and after breakfast.

Damage to the anus can also result in leakage. For example, stretching of the anal opening is a recognized treatment for hemorrhoids, but if it is done over-vigorously it can allow leakage. Women can develop the problem if the anal muscle is damaged by a tear, or occasionally by the episiotomy cut, made during childbirth. Damage to the *pudendal nerve* can also occur during childbirth, and result in incontinence. If you first noticed fecal incontinence after having a baby, see your doctor – a surgical operation to repair the damage often gives good results. Fecal leakage is also quite common in the elderly, because the anal muscle becomes weaker with age.

USEFUL CONTACTS

International Foundation for Functional Gastrointestinal Disorders
IFFGD, PO Box 17864, Milwaukee, WI 53217
1-888-964-2001
Email IFFGD at iffgd@iffgd.org

The American Gastroenterological Association has put up Irritable Bowel Syndrome in its public section
American Gastroenterological Association
National Office
7910 Woodmont Avenue, Suite 700
Bethesda, MD 20814
301-654-2055 fax: 301-654-5920
AGA Home Page: http://www.gastro.org
Email: member@gastro.org

genital warts

Genital warts are caused by a virus, HPV (*human papillomavirus*). HPV is caught during sexual contact with someone who is already infected with it. A man may not actually know that he has a wart, because it may be hidden inside the hole (urethral opening). Also, a woman can have a wart on the cervix (i.e. deep inside the vagina) which she doesn't know about.

Although you can catch the virus by sexual contact with someone who carries it but has no warts (15–40% of under 40s are carriers of HPV, though they are less common in older people), infection is more likely from someone who has warts. This is because the surface of a wart is teeming with the virus. After infection, warts can develop 3 weeks to 8 months later, so don't assume that you caught them from a recent sexual contact.

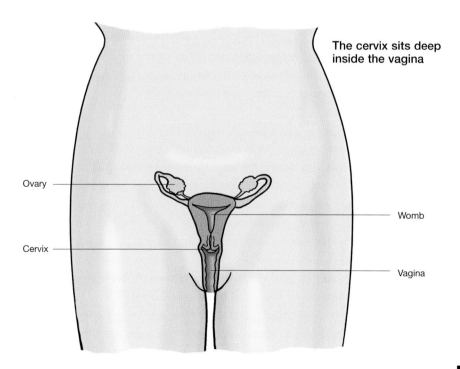

The cervix sits deep inside the vagina

Ovary

Womb

Cervix

Vagina

In women

Genital warts usually occur around the opening of the vagina (vulva). They may occur in the folds of skin alongside the vaginal opening, or between the vagina and the anus and around the anal opening.

If you feel inside the vagina (use two fingers) as high as you can, you will probably be able to feel your cervix. It feels like the tip of your nose, but has a dip in the middle. A pimple on the cervix could be a wart (see page 96), though it would be unusual to have warts on the cervix without having any at the opening of the vagina. If you do feel any pimples on the cervix you could ask your doctor to check them for you, or alternatively you could go to a clinic. Doctors at these clinics are used to looking at the cervix and answering any queries you might have. You do not need a referral from your doctor, but can simply call for an appointment yourself.

If you think you may have genital warts, or if a partner tells you he has or has had warts, go to a health clinic for a check. This is important, because HPV may agitate the cells of the cervix and encourage pre-cancerous changes.

Any woman who has had genital warts, or whose partner has genital warts, needs to have a cervical smear every year. The warts themselves are treated by freezing or by applying trichloroacetic acid or podophyllin. These treatments are tedious (as they have to be done once or twice a week), may cause soreness, podophyllin has to be washed off at a set time after the application, and it may take months for the warts to go. A newer treatment – podophyllotoxin – is applied twice daily for 3 days every week and is slightly more effective, but causes more soreness.

In men

Genital warts often occur just under the foreskin, but can be anywhere on the penis, on the scrotum, in the groins or around the anus. On the scrotum or shaft of the penis, they usually resemble the ordinary warts that occur on the hands. Under the foreskin and round the anus they are usually a shiny pinkish-white. A lone wart may also occur inside the opening of the urethra (the passage for urine and semen); here it will be a pinkish colour and may look speckled. An individual may have dozens of warts, or just one or two.

Don't try to treat warts in the genital area with any of the wart lotions you can buy from the pharmacist; these are for use on the hands only. Genital warts on the penis are treated by dabbing on podophyllin or podophyllotoxin solution or trichloracetic acid; you cannot buy these from a pharmacist, so you need to see a doctor. The clinic

Genital warts and your female partner

- Your female partner will need a check-up for warts and a cervical smear, because HPV can irritate the cells on the cervix (neck of the womb) and increase the risk of cervical cancer.

- If you are in an ongoing relationship, tell your partner about the warts, if she has not already noticed them, and urge her to visit a clinic (see page 9). She may be shocked and reluctant to go, but the staff there will be very nice to her. If she refuses to go, urge her to see her doctor for a cervical smear at least.

- If you are no longer in a relationship with the person who probably gave you the warts, discuss the situation with the counselors (health advisers) at the clinic.

- You should avoid sexual intercourse or use condoms for 12 weeks after the warts have gone. This allows time for your partner to be checked, and also for you to be sure that the warts really have been eliminated. The exception is if you and your partner have been together, without any other partners, for a long time and have not been using condoms previously; in this situation she probably has the HPV already, even if she has no warts.

will do tests for other sexually transmitted diseases as well as treating the warts; 1 in 5 people with genital warts have another infection which they are probably unaware of. The treatment can be quite lengthy – the lotion may have to be applied two or three times a week for several weeks – but most clinics will supply a treatment pack for you to continue the treatment yourself at home. Some clinics treat large warts by freezing (cryotherapy) or electrocautery (burning them off).

hairiness in women

- 25% of young women have noticeable facial hair
- After menopause, the face becomes hairier, while the rest of the body's hair is slowly lost
- 10% of 65-year-old women have noticeable chin hair

Excess hair (*hirsutism*) in women often appears in the places where men have body hair – such as the upper lip and chin, the chest (including around the nipples), the tops of the shoulders and the lower abdomen. Women often worry that this means that they have male hormones and are not fully female.

In fact, all women have a small amount of the 'male' hormone, testosterone, circulating in their bodies. It is produced mainly by the adrenal glands which are situated over the kidneys. If the skin is extra sensitive to it, testosterone encourages hair growth on the upper lip, chin, chest, lower abdomen. The hormone levels are normal; the problem is that the skin is too sensitive to testosterone. Women with this problem gradually develop more body hair from puberty until menopause, after which the amount of body hair slowly lessens – except for facial hair which continues to increase.

There are many reasons for this extra sensitivity to testosterone. Often, it simply runs in the family and mother or aunts may have had the same problem. Some drugs can be responsible, particularly phenobarbitone and phenytoin taken to control epilepsy. Long-term steroids (taken for conditions such as arthritis or inflammatory bowel disease) and cyclosporin (taken for psoriasis, dermatitis or arthritis) can also cause extra hair growth.

In some women, the level of male hormone is too high. This is usually caused by cysts on the ovary (a condition called *polycystic ovary syndrome*). There are usually other symptoms as well as excess hair. Polycystic ovary syndrome sometimes runs in families. It is diagnosed by blood tests and, usually, an ultrasound scan of the ovaries. It can be treated by drugs. Women with polycystic ovary syndrome are often obese, and the hirsutism improves if they lose weight. Very occasionally, a tumor of the ovaries or adrenal gland is responsible for the excess male hormones.

Symptoms of polycystic ovary syndrome

- Usually develops in the late teens or early twenties
- Excess hair
- Missing or irregular periods, or periods stop altogether (but periods may be normal)
- Acne and greasy hair
- Difficulty getting pregnant

What you can do

- Lose weight if you are overweight. This may greatly improve the problem.
- Bleaching is a good way of disguising upper lip hairs, which are usually not very long.
- Plucking, waxing or sugaring will deal with the problem temporarily. Plucking is not a good idea for the face because it can easily cause scarring. In waxing, strips of hot wax are placed over the hairy area and pulled off, taking the hairs with them. This is painful, and difficult to use on the face. Sugaring is similar, but uses a special sugar paste obtainable from pharmacies.
- Shaving will need to be done every day. In spite of the old wives' tale, it does not make the hairs grow back more quickly, but they will be stubbly – so may be noticeable if shaving is not repeated daily.
- Electrolysis is probably the best method of getting rid of the unwanted hair permanently. However, it may take months or years of treatment before all the unwanted hairs are destroyed. A fine needle is inserted into the hair root, which is then destroyed by one of the following methods.
- With needle diathermy, high-frequency radio waves destroy the hair root in a few seconds, and the hair is then plucked out. A new hair should not form.
- With galvanism, a low-voltage electrical current is applied to the needle for about 2 minutes. This causes the release of sodium hydroxide around the hair root, destroying it by chemical action.

Treatment can be uncomfortable. It is important that you use a qualified practitioner. Check that the practitioner uses new, disposable (not simply re-sterilized) needles. Home kits for electrolysis are not a good idea; the current used is too low to destroy the hair root, so the effect is similar to plucking.

How your doctor can help

See your doctor if any of the following apply:

- you have any of the symptoms of polycystic ovary syndrome, such as periods becoming irregular or stopping altogether
- you are taking any drugs that might be responsible
- excess hair starts to appear suddenly in adult life
- no one else in your family has excess hair
- you are having to spend a lot of money on electrolysis
- you are depressed and worried by your appearance.

If polycystic ovary syndrome is a possibility, your doctor will refer you to an endocrinologist (hormone specialist). The drug treatment for polycystic ovary syndrome is effective, especially if you also lose weight; greasy skin and acne clear up in about 6 weeks but it can take 12–18 months for maximum improvement in the hirsutism.

If there is no hormone abnormality, and the hirsutism happens simply because your skin is especially sensitive to testosterone, your doctor may prescribe the combined oral contraceptive pill. About 1 in 10 women will see an improvement. If this does not help, your doctor may decide to try a combination of cyproterone acetate and ethinyloestradiol (Dianette), which stops testosterone having an effect on the skin. It will take about 3 months before there is any improvement, and 12–18 months for the full effect. After this, the drug is stopped. Hair may regrow about 6 months later, in which case another course of the drug can be given.

Some hospital dermatology departments provide electrolysis treatment, but this is usually available only for individuals with a great deal of excess hair, or who are particularly distressed by it.

hairy backs

"I've got more hair than other men –
even my back is very hairy. I feel like an ape"

- Research among medical students in the US found that 45% of male medical students were very hairy, compared with 10% of the general population
- In Kerala, in southern India, research among medical and engineering students and manual laborers found that the students had more body hair than the laborers; the top six in the class of engineering students were far hairier than the bottom eight
- A study of 117 male members of the brainy society Mensa (you have to have an IQ of over 140 to join) showed that Mensa members had a tendency to thicker body hair – and the most intelligent had hair on their backs as well as on their chests

Some women find hairiness very attractive. Hairiness is something to be proud of – hairy men are more intelligent. Hairy chests and backs are more likely to be found among the highly educated than in the general population. However, there are also very intelligent men with little or no body hair. Einstein had hardly any body hair!

headache during sex

"Sex gives me a headache – and my partner assumes it's the old avoidance ploy"

Headaches during sex sound like a joke, but they aren't funny to anyone who experiences them. Mysteriously, the headache may occur on some occasions but not on others, even with the same sexual technique. Sexual intercourse, or just masturbation, may bring on the pain. These headaches can occur at all ages and in both men and women, although they are three times more common in men. Interestingly, they tend to occur during male, but not female, orgasm, and during female but not male masturbation. They are also more common in people who already suffer from migraines.

Why the headache occurs
Sex can cause two sorts of headache.
- As sexual excitement increases, there is often a dull, cramping, tight feeling at the back of the head. This is probably due to excessive contraction of the muscles of the neck.
- At the moment of orgasm there can be a sudden, severe pain. This is probably due to contraction of some of the small blood vessels in the brain, similar to migraine, and in fact half the people with this type of headache are also migraine sufferers. This pain generally lasts less than an hour, but may be gone in 10 minutes or linger for a few hours. It usually has a throbbing quality.

Some people have only one of these headaches, but many people have both, so they experience a headache that increases with sexual excitement, and culminates in an explosive headache at orgasm.

Another cause of headache during sex is Viagra (sildenafil) – a pill for the treatment of impotence. Headache is one of its side-effects.

What you can do about it

Most people find they are more prone to these headaches when they are:

- tired or under stress
- attempting intercourse for the second or third time in close succession
- using an uncomfortable or strenuous position.

Try to avoid these situations! If you mainly have the dull headache at the back of the neck, make a deliberate effort to relax your neck muscles. This usually relieves it. If you suffer from the severe headache at orgasm, see your doctor who will be able to check that there is no serious reason and may be able to prescribe a drug such as propranolol to prevent it.

impotence

Myths about impotence

- 'Impotence is uncommon'. This is untrue – most men simply don't talk about it. A survey sponsored by the drug company Pharmacia & Upjohn found that more than 1 in 4 of the UK male population over the age of 16 have experienced erectile disorder to some degree. Of these, over half experienced the problem as one-off incidents and a quarter suffer erectile disorder most or all of the time. There are probably 20 million impotent men in the US, and 2 million in the UK
- 'Impotence is usually psychological'. This is an old-fashioned view: impotence is most commonly due to a physical cause
- 'Testosterone injections/patches are the main cure for impotence'. Testosterone is of use only in the uncommon situation where there is a proven shortage of testosterone

Impotence (also called erectile failure or erectile dysfunction) means that the man cannot achieve or maintain an erection of the penis sufficient for sexual intercourse. He may often have a normal sex drive. It can occur at any age, but becomes more common with increasing age. However, 40% of 90-year-olds are able to have a normal erection.

What happens during an erection

The penis contains three long cylinders – the erectile tissue. Two of the cylinders lie side-by-side while the third lies beneath them. The urethra, which is the urine and sperm channel, runs through this lower cylinder. Sexual excitement causes the cylinders to fill with blood – as they swell, so the penis becomes erect. And as the erectile tissue swells, it squeezes the veins in the penis. These veins normally drain blood away from the penis, so the squeezing actions prevents blood flowing away and keeps the penis erect. After orgasm and ejaculation these events go into reverse, and the penis becomes limp again.

How the system fails (impotence)

A few years ago it was assumed that most cases of impotence were due to psychological reasons. Now more is known about the blood supply to the penis, and it

The penis

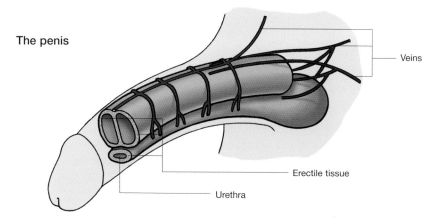

Veins

Erectile tissue

Urethra

is recognized that physical problems are often responsible. For example, the nerves to the spongy tissue can be damaged by diabetes, and blood flow can be damaged by vascular disease, or the veins may leak blood out instead of being effectively compressed.

Psychological factors can, of course, cause impotence. These include:

- guilt
- depression
- losing interest in your partner
- a partner who finds intercourse painful
- low self-esteem
- fear of not performing well.

Often both physical and psychological factors are involved. A physical problem impairs erections, and you then become so preoccupied with the question 'Can I maintain my erection this time?' that sexual arousal becomes impossible. Anxiety actually has the physical effect of contracting the muscles of the erectile tissue, preventing blood entering the penis and allowing the blood to drain away.

How to approach your doctor

According to *Men's Health* magazine, 'on the Richter scale of embarrassment, impotence comes near the top'. This is the problem men least like discussing with their doctor, but it is of course the one problem that the doctor will not be able to guess that you have, unless you mention it. When you do manage to discuss it you will probably find that your doctor is surprisingly matter-of-fact about it. In fact, treatments for impotence have now been so much in the news that more and more people are discussing the problem with their doctor, so he or she will not be surprised. Impotence, or erectile failure, is a standard medical problem that doctors are now trained to deal with. It is possible that you have a local specialist hospital clinic.

If you keep avoiding the issue with your doctor there are two other possible approaches. Your partner could have a preliminary discussion with the doctor to pave the way. Or you could write to your doctor, marking the envelope 'Confidential' and explaining that you have been too embarrassed to mention the problem but would like an appointment to discuss it, if possible at the end of a day when the doctor would have more time.

Even if you convince yourself that the problem is due to stress, see your doctor. You may be wrong, and even if you are right your doctor should be able to help.

Questions to ask yourself

- *Is it really an erection problem?* Or is the actual problem premature ejaculation (see page 71) or a lack of sexual desire (see page 122)?
- *Can you achieve an erection by masturbation but not with your partner, and do you still sometimes wake with an erection?* If the answers are 'yes', a psychological reason, such as stress or depression, is likely.
- *Did loss of erections come on suddenly, or have erections gradually been failing over a long period of time?* Erectile failure which comes on suddenly is usually psychological; physical causes usually have a more gradual onset.
- *Have you been under extra stress lately?* If so, is there any way you can lessen the stress in your life?
- *Are you taking any drugs that might be responsible?* If so, ask your doctor for alternatives.
- *Are you drinking too much?* Blood alcohol concentrations of up to about 25 mg/100 ml improve erections slightly, but when the level reaches about 40 mg/100 ml erection is inhibited. In some people, only one or two drinks is enough to raise the blood alcohol to this level. Heavy drinking over a long period can cause erectile failure because of nerve damage.
- *Have you noticed anything else wrong?* For example: Peyronie's disease, where the penis develops a lump and often kinks (page 111), can cause impotence; tightness of the foreskin (see page 117) can prevent full erections; enlargement of the breasts or loss of body hair might mean a hormonal problem.

Drugs that can cause erectile failure (impotence)

- Cimetidine (for duodenal ulcer)
- Some drugs for hypertension (for example, thiazide diuretics, methyldopa, beta-blockers)
- Finasteride (for prostate enlargement or baldness)
- Phenothiazines (for some psychiatric conditions)
- Alcohol
- Drugs used for prostate cancer (for example, some GnRH analogues and anti-androgens)
- Antidepressants

- *Who is really bothered by the problem – you or your partner?* Talk to your partner about what each of you wants from sex. As sex counselor Susie Hayman says, "It's amazing how many people just lie there wishing their partner was a mindreader."

What your doctor can do

Your doctor will consider whether impotence is the result of some medical condition or any drugs that you are taking. Impotence can also result from depression and from relationship problems, so be prepared for some talk along these lines. However, most doctors believe that there is no point in deep psychoanalytical-type discussions; they prefer to do a few simple investigations and then deal with the problem in a practical way.

If a prescribed drug might be the cause, your doctor will probably be able to change to another pill and this will usually solve the problem. If it doesn't, it may be that the

Conditions that can cause erectile failure (impotence)

- Diabetes
- Hypertension
- Vascular disease
- Severe liver disease
- Thyroid disease
- Neurological conditions (for example, spinal injury, multiple sclerosis)
- Depression
- Peyronie's disease (see page 111)
- After some prostate operations (especially radical prostatectomy)
- Renal failure

Tests usually carried out

● Blood or urine glucose, to check for diabetes.

● Blood testosterone (male hormone) level can be measured. However, it is unusual for impotence to be caused by a low testosterone level, so the result is usually normal. The exception is when there has been a reduced sex drive for some time before any problem with erections; in this situation a testosterone test is worthwhile.

● Blood prolactin level is sometimes measured if erectile failure was preceded by a reduced sex drive; a high level of this hormone is extremely rare but may be associated with impotence, and can be an indicator of other diseases.

drug was not responsible. Alternatively, you may have developed a psychological block – 'fear of failure' – which may take time and counselling to overcome.

If stress, depression or a relationship problem seems to be a factor, counselling and/or antidepressant medication may be the answer. If you require an antidepressant do not worry that you will be hooked for life; these drugs are given for a limited period to kick-start you out of your depression. However, they may take several weeks to work, and some antidepressants can themselves impair erections.

What a urology/impotence clinic can do

Some doctors have set up special impotence clinics seeing patients from their own and other practices. Otherwise, your doctor will refer you to a urologist. The urologist can provide the following ways of obtaining an erection, and will discuss these with you to see which would suit you best. Avoid the private clinics you see advertised in the media.

Penile rings (for example, Rapport RLS) are helpful for people who can get an erection but find that it does not last.

Injecting alprostadil into the penis is the treatment favored by many specialists. Alprostadil (as in, for example, Caverject) is a synthetic version of prostaglandin E1. This chemical relaxes the tiny muscles of the erectile tissue while increasing blood supply. It is injected 10–30 minutes before intercourse. The doctor will inject the first dose and assess your erection to find the correct dose for you, and will show you how to inject yourself. The injection should produce an erection lasting about half an hour. Occasionally a prolonged response develops (priapism). If this is the case you should consult your doctor after 4–6 hours. If you have a needle phobia or cannot easily see the penis, an automatic system is available (Autoject 2.25). One in six people experiences some pain in the penis following the injection, and there might also be some bruising.

Injecting the penis with moxisylyte (Erecnos) is a newer treatment that has been under study in the US and available in the UK since September 1997. For an erection to happen, the tiny muscles in the spongy part of the penis must relax to allow blood in. Most of the time, when the penis is flaccid, these tiny muscles are kept contracted by a body chemical called noradrenaline. Moxisylyte stops the noradrenaline from working, so the tiny muscles relax, blood flows in, and the penis becomes erect. Only 1 in 100 men experiences pain with moxisylyte, though this treatment does not work for everyone. Of 300 men using it at home, about two-thirds said it produced an erection adequate for sex.

MUSE (alprostadil pellet) has been under study in the U.S. and available in the UK since February 1998. MUSE stands for 'medicated urethral system for erection'. A small pellet of alprostadil, no bigger than a grain of rice, is inserted about 3 cm up the urethra, using a tiny plastic plunger. Although it is not an injection, some men find it painful, but this discomfort can be minimized by urinating beforehand. Another disadvantage is that it makes some men feel slightly dizzy. MUSE takes 5–10 minutes to work, and the erection lasts 30–60 minutes. It does not cause abnormally prolonged erections (priapism).

In the US, an alprostadil gel which is applied to the penis is being researched. The gel contains an additional ingredient to help absorption of the drug through the skin of the penis.

Vacuum devices consist of a plastic cylinder with a pump, which may be hand- or battery-operated. A special ring is placed around the cylinder, and the cylinder is then placed over the penis. The pump is activated to produce a vacuum inside the cylinder, sucking blood into the penis, which becomes erect. When the erection is sufficient, the ring is slipped off the cylinder on to the base of the penis, to maintain the erection. The erection lasts until the ring is removed. Vacuum devices are effective but they are cumbersome and some people find them off-putting because the penis, while erect, is often blue or mottled, and cold. They are supplied with an instruction video. The cost is about $200-300. Most companies allow a trial period with money returned if the device proves unsatisfactory. Side-effects such as bruising are uncommon.

Yohimbine tablets. Yohimbine comes from the bark of the *Pausinystalin yohimbe* tree, which for over a century has been thought to possess aphrodisiac qualities. Various trials have shown success rates of 30–70%, slightly better than the success rates from placebo (dummy) tablets.

Viagra (sildenafil) tablets. Viagra is a treatment for impotence, which is taken by mouth. It prevents the breakdown of some of the chemicals in the penis that are involved in erections, so it helps the normal erectile mechanism. A man taking Viagra becomes erect only with sexual stimulation – unlike the other treatments, which produce an erection whether or not the man is aroused. As the sex drive abates, so do the drug's effects. So, overall, it seems to provide a more natural erection than the other methods.

Viagra is taken 30–60 minutes before intercourse, and 88% of men using it report that it improves erections. Side-effects include headache, flushing, diarrhea, dizziness and abnormal vision. More worryingly, there have been reports of deaths from heart attacks in men using the drug. It is unclear whether they died because of an interaction between heart medication and Viagra, or whether unaccustomed sexual exertion was the real reason. Viagra should not be used by anyone taking nitrates (for angina), and should not be taken more than once a day.

Surgery to improve blood supply to the penis or to stop blood leaking from it back into the body is possible in certain cases. The results are often disappointing.

Surgical implants to stiffen the penis can be inserted if all else fails. There are several new types, which are much superior to those used just a few years ago. Some are inflatable, and these are much more natural when inflated and more easily concealed when deflated than in the past. These inflatables use a reservoir that is inserted beneath the abdominal muscle during a small operation. The reservoir is filled with salty water (saline). When you want an erection, you trigger a pump placed in the scrotum next to the testicle. This signal shifts fluid from the reservoir into the cylinders that have been inserted into the penis. An alternative to the inflatables is the 'malleable' (bendy) type, which maintains a constant erection using flexible rods that can be manipulated into a concealed position.

Both inflatable and bendy implants are expensive and require surgery, but are effective and most men who have implants are pleased with them. The inflatables and the malleable types are seen as equally successful, though one survey showed that female partners tend to prefer the inflatable type. The main problem with the inflatable type is fluid leakage (which occurs in about 3% of men over 3 years, and will need a further operation to correct the problem) and infection (which occurs in about 3–5% and usually means that the implant has to be removed).

USEFUL CONTACTS

Sexual Function Health Council
c/o American Foundation for Urologic Disease, Inc
1128 North Charles Street
Baltimore, MD 21201
(800) 433-4215
www.afud.org

Impotence Resource Center
Sexual Function Health Council
American Foundation for Urologic Disease
1128 N. Charles Street
Baltimore, Maryland 21201
(800) 433-4215
www.impotence.org

National Kidney and Urologic Diseases Information Clearinghouse
3 Information Way
Bethesda, MD 20892-3580
(301) 654-4415
www.niddk.nih.gov

American Diabetes Association National Center
1660 Duke Street
Alexandria, VA 22314
(800) 232-3472
www.diabetes.org

jock itch

"I can't help scratching my groin – it's so itchy"

Jock itch with a rash

Jock itch is usually an itchy rash in the fold of skin in the groin. Often the skin fold beneath the scrotum is affected as well. Usually the area is red and slightly scaly. It usually has a sharp border, demarcating it clearly from the unaffected skin. If you look closely at the border you may see small pimples. The rash spreads outwards, and as it does so the center may clear.

This is sometimes known as 'sweat rash', but it isn't caused by sweat. The actual cause is a *tinea* fungus, the same fungus that causes athlete's foot. In fact, jock itch is probably 'caught' from your own feet. Check between your toes for the red, scaly appearance of athlete's foot. Athlete's foot is very common in people who do a lot of sports, because it is easily caught from the floors of communal changing rooms and showers.

Although sweat doesn't cause the rash, the fungus does thrive in warm, moist, sweaty conditions, so you can help yourself by:

- not wearing tight underpants
- wearing 100% cotton underpants instead of synthetic fabrics
- drying yourself carefully in the groin and around the testicles after bathing or showering
- losing weight if you have a paunch
- looking after your feet (see page 157) to avoid athlete's foot.

Fungi also thrive on skin that is slightly damaged. One of the most common ways of damaging skin is by perfumes in soaps, shampoos and shower gels and by enzyme washing powders so:

- wash with an unperfumed soap

- if you wash your hair in the shower, don't let the foam run down your body into the groin creases
- don't use 'enzyme' or 'biological' washing powders for your underpants.

These self-help measures will discourage the fungus but probably won't eliminate it, so see your doctor for an antifungal cream.

Jock itch without a rash
Sometimes the groin area can be very itchy but there is no rash to be seen. In this case a fungal infection is unlikely. Probably your skin is very sensitive to soaps and perfumes, so follow the advice above.

lumps on the genitals

Women

The cervix

The main lump in the vagina is the cervix (neck of the womb). This projects into the far end of the vagina and is about 3 cm across. You can usually feel the cervix by inserting the first two fingers into the vagina and pushing upwards. It is easier to feel if you 'bear down' (contract your stomach muscles as if you are trying to open your bowels). The texture of the cervix is similar to the end of your nose, but it has a hole in the middle. In a woman who has not had a child, the hole is about the size of a pencil lead, but it is usually larger in women who have given birth. Menstrual blood passes through this hole from the womb into the vagina.

The cervix usually feels smooth, but sometimes pimples can be felt on it. These are usually small glands called *nabothian follicles*, and are normal.

Position of the cervix

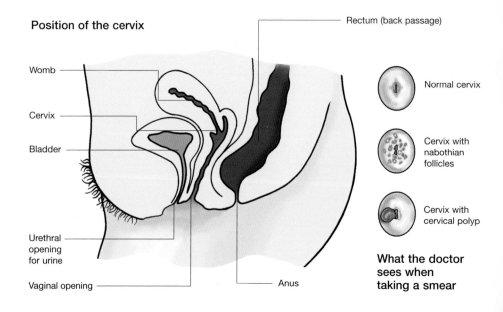

Womb

Cervix

Bladder

Urethral opening for urine

Vaginal opening

Rectum (back passage)

Anus

Normal cervix

Cervix with nabothian follicles

Cervix with cervical polyp

What the doctor sees when taking a smear

However, a pimple on the cervix could be a wart (see page 77), though it would be unusual to have warts on the cervix without having any at the opening of the vagina (vulva).

A small, soft lump which seems to be coming out of the hole in the cervix is probably a cervical polyp. This is not cancerous, but can bleed, especially after intercourse, so it is best to have it removed.

Small lumps in the vagina

The inside of the vagina can normally feel crinkly. This is because it is designed to stretch for intercourse and childbirth, so when it is not stretched the walls may have wrinkles. However, it is not normal to have distinct small lumps in the vagina. If you feel any, see your doctor or go to a health clinic because they could be warts (though it is unusual to have vaginal warts without any at the vulva).

Prolapse

A bulge in the vagina is probably a *prolapse*. The vagina rests between the bladder and rectum; the bladder lies in front of it and the rectum (back passage) lies behind. The bladder, vagina, cervix and rectum are held in position by muscles that stretch across the pelvis – the pelvic floor muscles. If these muscles are weak, the bladder and/or rectum can lean towards the vagina and press on it, or the womb may sag downwards.

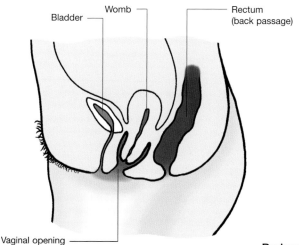

Bladder

Womb

Rectum (back passage)

Vaginal opening

Prolapse – the womb sags down

Symptoms of prolapse

- A leaning bladder is felt as a lump in the vagina, towards the front. Urine may leak on coughing or sneezing (stress incontinence, see page 167), and you may get bladder infections (such as cystitis).
- A leaning rectum is felt as a lump in the vagina, towards the back.
- If the cervix and womb are sagging down, the cervix can be felt quite near the opening of the vagina, rather than needing to push up with stretched fingers to feel it. It may be difficult to keep tampons in. The cervix can even sag down so far that it projects out of the vaginal opening. This can be alarming, because its pink color and its hole make it look similar to a penis.
- These symptoms are often worse at the end of a long day or after standing for a long time.
- All types of prolapse can cause problems during sex. Intercourse may be uncomfortable. You may have a loss of sensation, and find it difficult to have an orgasm. Air can be trapped in the vagina during sex, and then be expelled like a fart (*vaginal flatus*).

Treatment for prolapse is really surgery, but other measures may be of some benefit.

- Lose weight if you are obese. This will certainly help; excess weight puts pressure on the pelvic floor and makes the problem worse.
- Stop smoking if you have a smoker's cough; coughing puts pressure on the pelvic floor.
- Do pelvic floor exercises (see page 170). They will help leakage of urine due to prolapse.
- Hormone replacement therapy may possibly increase the strength of the vagina and pelvic floor, but there is no definite proof.
- Surgery is needed if prolapse is troublesome, particularly if it is causing incontinence of urine. The surgeon cuts away flabby parts of the vagina and strengthens the supporting tissues. It is important to tell the surgeon if you are still sexually active, so that the vagina is not made too narrow, or intercourse may later be uncomfortable.

Causes of prolapse

Weakness of the pelvic floor muscles
- Large babies
- Long labor, especially if forceps were needed
- Not having done pelvic floor exercises after childbirth
- Hysterectomy

Increased pressure
- Obesity
- Chronic chest problem (such as smoker's cough)

- A pessary is a special ring placed in the vagina to give support. Pessaries are made of plastic and are changed every 6 months. They are usually used as a stop-gap measure while waiting for an operation, or for women who cannot have surgery for any reason.

Lumps at the entrance to the vagina

In many women the entrance to the vagina normally feels lumpy. This lumpiness is the remains of the hymen which stretches across the entrance in young girls. The hymen is a thin piece of tissue with a hole to let menstrual blood flow out. The hole becomes enlarged during sports and by inserting tampons, and by sexual intercourse, but the remnants of the hymen can remain as irregular, firm lumpiness.

A woman who has given birth to a child, and who needed stitches afterwards, may be left with a lumpy scar at the vaginal opening.

Genital warts are increasingly common, and often occur around the vaginal entrance (see page 77).

Men

"Some lumps have appeared on my penis"

Sometimes we look at our bodies in a new light, and notice things that we have never seen before, and we think they are not normal. This often happens with the genital area, partly because it is not easy to compare with other people's. If you notice any new lumps or bumps, ask your doctor to check, or go to a clinic (see page 9). This is because any lumps might actually be warts or other conditions, which should be treated.

Lumps and bumps on the penis that are normal

Pearly penile papules are small lumps, about 1–2 mm across. They look like pimples and are all roughly the same size and shape. They are in a row around the margin of the head of the penis, and can be seen when the foreskin is pulled back. In some men they are hardly visible at all, and in others they are quite noticeable. They usually develop in the teens. People often worry that they are warts or an infection, and pick or squeeze them. In fact they are perfectly normal tiny glands. Leave them alone!

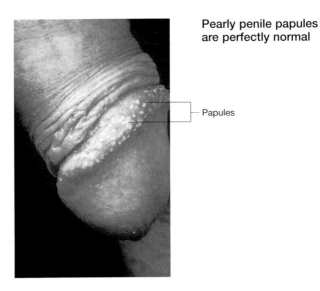

**Pearly penile papules
are perfectly normal**

— Papules

A lymphocele is a hard swelling that suddenly appears after sexual intercourse or masturbation. It is usually on the shaft of the penis, near the foreskin. It is caused by temporary blockage of the lymphatic channels at the margin of the head of the penis. It will go away on its own, and there are no after-effects.

Lumps and bumps on the penis that are not normal
Genital warts are very common (see page 77).

Molluscum contagiosum are pinkish-white round lumps, each about 1–5 mm in diameter. If you look at them very closely (ideally with a magnifying glass) you will see that each one has a dimple in its centre. This distinguishes them from warts. There may be just one molluscum, but usually there are between 5 and 20. They can occur on any part of the body, but are usually on the penis, upper thighs and lower abdomen. Although they are not warts, they are caused by a virus. They are caught by skin contact, usually sexual. (In women they tend to occur on the vaginal lips, upper thighs and lower abdomen.) They may appear 2 weeks to 6 months after infection has occurred.

   The treatment is rather odd. They tend to disappear if they are damaged in any way, so doctors often jab them with a needle or cocktail stick dipped into phenol or iodine. This treatment is painful, but it gets rid of them. Large ones are sometimes treated by freezing (*cryotherapy*).

Lichen nitidus is tiny, shiny, flat-topped, flesh-colored pimples which are difficult to distinguish from warts. The pimples are usually on the shaft of the penis and their cause is a mystery. They may remain the same for years, or may disappear of their own accord. They do not usually need any treatment.

Ulcers on the glans may be due to genital herpes, an infection caused by a virus, or, less commonly the ulcer may be a special form of skin cancer. If an ulcer or ulcers develop then you should consult your doctor without too much delay.

Lumps and bumps on the scrotum that are normal
Chicken-skin scrotum. It is normal for the skin of the scrotum to look like the skin of a plucked chicken. This is because the hair follicles on the scrotum are quite far apart and prominent, while the hairs themselves may not be very obvious.

Sebaceous cysts are swollen, blocked grease glands that look like yellowish pimples. They often occur on the skin of the scrotum, and there may be a dozen or more. The skin contains millions of glands that make grease to keep the skin waterproof and in good condition. The openings of these glands easily become blocked, so they become distended with grease. For some reason, the skin of the scrotum seems particularly susceptible to this problem. They are harmless, but if they become infected (red and sore) or you don't like the look of them, a clinic will be able to treat them.

Angiokeratoma of Fordyce are tiny, bright red blood-blisters. They usually occur on the scrotum, and there may be lots of them. They are quite common in the late teens, and are normal. Their only problem is that they can be itchy, and may bleed if you scratch them.

Lumps and bumps on the scrotum that are not normal
Genital warts (see page 77)

Varicoceles are the result of swelling of the veins around the testis. Most commonly varicoceles occur on the left. They often feel like a 'bag of worms' and are more noticeable on standing. They are generally harmless but may cause testicular ache or reduced fertility because of abnormally high temperatures around the testicles.

Lump in the scrotum. A lump attached to the testicle may sometimes be felt through the skin of the scrotum. While many of these are harmless cysts, occasionally a lump may be due to the development of testicular cancer. If you do find a lump in your scrotum you should consult your doctor who will usually refer you to a urologist. Most tumors of the testes are curable (that is, they don't come back), if removed early.

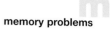

memory problems

*"My memory is much worse than it was
– I think I'm getting Alzheimer's"*

If you notice that your memory is poor, it is natural to think of the worst explanation – Alzheimer's disease. In actual fact, there is usually another reason and the problem is usually temporary. The most common cause is depression. With depression, many of the mental processes are slowed, and memory is particularly affected. Unfortunately, worry about memory loss can worsen the depression, producing a vicious circle:

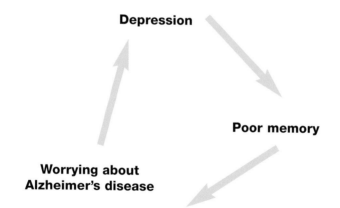

Depression

Poor memory

**Worrying about
Alzheimer's disease**

Another common cause is stress. Almost any worry or stressful life event can affect our ability to store memories and recall them. When the problem is resolved, or time has healed the pain, memory becomes as efficient as it was before.

Of course, a failing memory does occur with Alzheimer's disease. Alzheimer's is mainly a disease of the elderly. About 1% of people in their 60s, 20% of those over 85 years and 30% of those over 90 years of age are affected.

Stressful life events that can affect memory

- Work-related problems
- Divorce or other relationship problems
- Being charged with a crime
- Being involved in litigation
- Bereavement

What you can do

- Try to work out whether you have had an unusual amount of stress recently, or if there is any possibility that you are depressed. For example, has there been any change in your sleep pattern? Sleeping a great deal less or more than in the past, difficulty getting to sleep or waking early in the morning are all pointers to depression or anxiety.
- Ask a friend or member of your family whether they have noticed your memory has deteriorated. As a general rule, if memory loss is due to anxiety or depression, people notice and worry about it themselves; if it is due to Alzheimer's, other people are much more aware of it than the sufferer.

What your doctor can do

Depression can creep up so gradually that you may not be aware that you are suffering from it, so your doctor will first assess whether or not you are depressed. If so, antidepressant medication would be the most appropriate treatment, and would restore your memory. The improvement might not be immediate, because antidepressant drugs can take several months to have an effect. Your doctor could also help you to identify stresses or problems that may be affecting your memory, and could advise on coping strategies.

If you or your doctor cannot work out the reason for your memory problem, he or she could refer you to a memory clinic. Memory clinics assess whether or not you have a memory impairment and what the cause might be. They also teach strategies to improve the ability to acquire new information and to consolidate and recall facts.

nipples

"My nipples don't stick out; they look like dimples. I can't go topless on the beach, and I'm worried I won't be able to breast-feed"

Inverted nipples

Most women's nipples protrude about 5–10 mm, and become about 10 mm longer and 2–3 mm wider during sexual arousal. Some women have nipples that are flat, but become erect during sexual arousal or when a baby is sucking on the nipple. Nipples that are tucked into the breast, instead of being flat or sticking out, are called *inverted nipples.* Both nipples may be inverted, or just one. If your nipples have been inverted for as long as you can remember, it is nothing to worry about. It is just the way you are, and a lot of women are the same. A survey of 3000 women attending an antenatal clinic found that 10% had inverted nipples.

Breast-feeding shouldn't be too much of a problem if your nipples become erect in the cold or when you are sexually aroused. It will be harder for the baby to draw the nipple into the back of its mouth, so breast-feeding will require some patience, but eventually the baby's strong sucking will draw the nipple out. You will be able to help by applying an ice cube wrapped in a flannel to the nipple beforehand and by stroking the areola (the pink area round the nipple).

If stimulation doesn't make the nipple protrude, breast-feeding may be more difficult. During the last 6–8 weeks of pregnancy you may be able to encourage the nipples to stick out by wearing breast shields under your bra. These are small devices which press gently on the breast around the nipple. They are quite comfortable. They are worn for 1 or 2 hours at first, and the time is gradually increased.

Even if you don't intend to breast-feed you may wish to have protruding nipples. Young girls often have flat nipples, and in some women (especially if their periods didn't start until late) they remain flat until the early 20s. So if you are young there is a possibility that they may gradually start to protrude. Otherwise, you could try stroking the areola with warm hands for a few minutes each day to bring the nipple out. You could also try wearing breast shields. Don't wear them for too long at first, otherwise the breasts may become sore, and don't continue wearing them for more than 6 weeks.

If these measures do not work, and your nipples are really distressing you, it is possible to have a small operation to make the nipples protrude. This involves a small incision on each side of the nipple, and the cutting of some ducts and tissue. The drawback is that some women cannot breast-feed after this operation.

A nipple that suddenly becomes inverted can be a sign of a cancer underneath it, so you should see your doctor straight away.

Hairy nipples

"My nipples have hairs growing round them"

Coarse, dark hairs around the nipple are quite common. You can pull them out with tweezers, but this can cause irritation because the skin round the nipple is very sensitive. It is probably better simply to cut them off close to the skin. This is easier if you hold the end of the hair with tweezers to keep it taut. The hairs will grow again, so you will have to cut them off again from time to time.

Hairs round the nipple are nothing to worry about unless you have excess hairiness on other parts of the body (see page 80) and your periods are irregular. If this is the case, you may have ovarian cysts, so you need to see your doctor.

oral sex

"Is oral sex safe?"

Oral sex can take place in various ways. For example:

- the woman can stimulate the man's penis with her mouth and tongue *(fellatio, blow job)*
- the man can stimulate the woman's vulva and clitoris with his tongue *(cunnilingus)*
- one partner can stimulate the area round the other partner's anus *(rimming)* with his or her tongue.

It is possible to catch infections by oral sex but, in general, the chances are probably lower than with penetrative sex. The risks also depend on whether you are the partner performing oral sex, or the partner who is having it done to them.

Risks to the partner performing oral sex

It is quite easy to catch gonorrhea throat infection by performing oral sex on a man who has it. He will have a discharge from the urethral opening (the hole at the end of the penis), and this discharge will be teeming with gonorrhea bacteria. Unfortunately, the discharge is not always very noticeable, so neither partner may be aware that he has the infection. Alternatively, he may have noticed a discharge previously, but may have assumed that the problem had cured itself. The message is that you should not perform oral sex on a man who has a discharge, or has recently had one which was not treated.

It is not a good idea to perform oral sex on a man who has genital warts. These may not be obvious, so check the margin of the head of the penis (glans) under the foreskin, and just inside the urethral opening. Although the risk is not great, a woman can develop a wart on the roof of her mouth as a result of oral sex. The wart may take weeks or even months to appear. If you develop one, go to your local health clinic (see page 9).

Similarly, it is possible for a man to develop a wart on his lips from performing oral sex on a woman who has genital warts. If this happens to you, a health clinic is the place to go.

There is very little clear evidence on the risk of catching HIV by oral sex. The body fluids of a person who has HIV (including semen and the natural fluids that lubricate the vagina) will contain the virus. So HIV can enter the mouth of the person performing oral sex, which might lead to infection if he or she happens to have any sores or cracks in the mouth. The risk is likely to be greater for a woman performing oral sex on a man than the other way round. Withdrawing the penis before the man's orgasm (ejaculation) would lessen the risk; however, when a man is sexually aroused, small amounts of semen leak out of the urethra before ejaculation so infection could still occur. Although the risk is low, it is not absolutely safe, and oral sex with someone who might be HIV-positive cannot be described as 'safe sex'. Some experts say you should avoid mouth-to-genital contact unless you are very sure that your partner is HIV-negative. Otherwise, avoid brushing your teeth beforehand, because this could open up cracks in the gum which would make it easier for the virus to enter.

Swallowing semen during oral sex is not harmful. It is unlikely to increase the risk of HIV because the stomach contains acid which destroys HIV.

Rimming (licking around the anus) is not recommended. The lower bowel contains many bacteria and viruses, which could enter the mouth, even if the anal area is washed beforehand. There is some evidence that Kaposi's sarcoma, the unpleasant skin cancer that sometimes accompanies AIDS, is an infection from the bowel acquired in this way.

Condoms for oral sex

If a man wears a condom, his partner is unlikely to catch anything by performing oral sex on him. If you are concerned about infection during oral sex, but don't like the idea of condoms because of their off-putting rubbery taste, try flavored ones. Textured, knobbed or ribbed condoms are not suitable for oral sex, because they can make the mouth sore (see page 60).

The partner who is having oral sex done to them

Apart from being bitten, catching genital herpes is the main risk. If your partner has a cold sore on his or her face or lip, don't let him or her perform oral sex on you. Cold sores are also infectious at the tingling stage before the sore has developed. If your partner has recurrent cold sores, he or she will recognize this tingling feeling, and should avoid performing oral sex until the sore has healed completely. Likewise, don't offer oral sex if you have a cold sore or think you might be getting one.

Contact between your genitals and the mouth of someone with HIV means that your genitals are in contact with their saliva, which will contain the HIV virus. The concentration of HIV in the saliva would be very small and there would probably be a very low risk of infection – but it would not be absolutely safe. The partner performing oral sex should avoid teeth brushing beforehand, because this can make the gums bleed and increase the amount of HIV in the saliva.

USEFUL CONTACTS

The National Herpes Hotline (919 361-8488) is operated by the American Social Health Association as part of the Herpes Resource Center (HRC). The hotline, which currently answers more than 30,000 calls a year, provides free counseling on herpes and offers referrals. The hotline is open from 9 a.m. to 7 p.m., EST, Monday through Friday. ASHA coordinates over 80 local support groups, called HELP Groups, in the U.S., Canada, and Australia.

American Social Health Association
PO Box 13827
Research Triangle Park, NC 27709
(919) 361-8400 Voice (919) 361-8425 Fax
www.ashastd.org

The National AIDS Treatment Advocacy Project - NATAP is an organization dedicated to educating the diverse communities affected by HIV on the latest HIV treatments and advocating on treatment and policy issues for people with HIV.
580 Broadway, Suite 403
New York, NY 10012
212-219-0106
www.natap.org

National Women's Health Information Center provides access to thousands of publications and organizations with information on hundreds of health topics:

8550 Arlington Blvd.
Fairfax, VA 22031.
1-800-994-WOMAN (1-800-994-9662)
www.4women.gov

penis

Bending

"My penis is crooked, especially when it's erect"

A condition called *Peyronie's disease* occasionally develops in men, in which the penis becomes crooked when it is erect. This can make sexual intercourse difficult, if not impossible. The condition is named after Dr François Gigot de la Peyronie who wrote about it in 1743, but it has probably been around for much longer; sculptures dating from the 6th century BC depict angulated erect penises. Another, much less common, cause is severe hypospadias which is discussed on page 115.

Peyronie's disease most commonly occurs in men aged 50–60, but it can occur in young men and in old age. The cause is thickening of the fibrous tissue in the penis on one side. This means that during an erection one side of the penis cannot lengthen, and the penis will bend. The direction of the bend depends on the position of the thickening (which can often be felt as a lump or lumps when the penis is flaccid). If it is on the top of the penis, the erection tends to curve upwards. If it is on either side, the penis will bend towards the side which is thickened.

When the condition develops, men with Peyronie's disease find that the thickened area is painful when the penis is erect. Those who have had the condition for a long time feel no pain but sometimes have difficulty achieving an erection (perhaps because the lumpiness is obstructing blood flow in the penis).

What causes Peyronie's disease?

No one knows why the thickening occurs, but it is not a cancerous condition, nor is it the result of sexually transmitted disease or of any odd previous sexual practices. There seems to be a link with some other conditions. For example, men with Peyronie's disease are quite likely to have Dupuytren's contracture, a thickening of fibrous tissue in the palm of the hand. They are also quite likely to have raised blood pressure; some doctors think that the blood pressure itself might be responsible for the penis problem, while others blame the drugs used to treat blood pressure (particularly beta-blockers).

Treatments

There is no need to feel embarrassed about discussing the problem with your doctor, because doctors are very familiar with the condition. If it is only mild, and doesn't cause any inconvenience, it can be left alone. In the past, the most common treatment was steroid injection into the thickening, but this is now less popular. Tablets of vitamin E 800 mg/day or potassium aminobenzoate (Potaba) 12 g/day may produce some improvement; you will need a doctor's prescription.

The most effective treatment is a simple operation to correct the deformity. Some tissue is cut away from the opposite side to balance out the thickened area. After the operation the erect penis will be straight but 1–3 cm shorter than before.

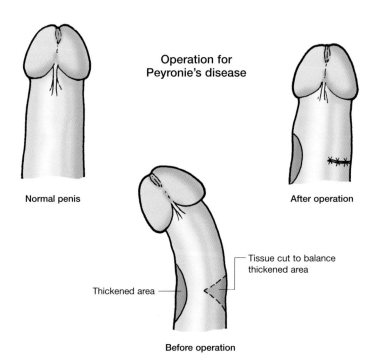

Operation for
Peyronie's disease

Normal penis

After operation

Tissue cut to balance
thickened area

Thickened area

Before operation

Discharge

*"I have some discharge from the hole at the end of my penis.
Is it likely to be serious?"*

The hole at the end of the penis is the opening of the urethra (the tube for urine and semen). Discharge is usually a sign of infection in the urethra. The most common are *non-specific urethritis,* or NSU for short, and gonorrhea.

NSU

This causes a discharge that is usually clear, and is worse in the mornings. You may find it uncomfortable to pass urine, and you may feel irritation along the urethra inside the penis.

NSU is caught during sex. Several types of bacteria may be responsible, though about half of cases are caused by *Chlamydia* and about 20% are caused by *Ureaplasma*. These bacteria do not cause a discharge in women, or any other symptoms in the early stages, so most women don't know that they have an infection.

In women, *Chlamydia* can travel upwards into the Fallopian tubes (the tubes that carry the eggs from the ovaries to the womb), and can eventually affect the tubes, making the woman infertile. For this reason you need treatment, so that you do not pass the infection on to a female partner.

Gonorrhea is caused by *Gonococcus* bacteria. Like NSU, it is caught during sex, and causes a discharge and pain when you pass urine. The discharge can be any color – yellow, green, white, cloudy or clear. The symptoms may be so slight that you hardly notice them, or there may be a lot of discharge. Gonorrhea can spread to the testicles, causing pain, swelling and redness. As with NSU, the woman you caught it from was probably unaware that she was infected; only 10–20% of women with gonorrhea have a discharge.

Inflammation

Occasionally, the urethra can become inflamed without there being any infection. For example, if you poke anything up the urethra you can damage the lining, which will become inflamed and cause a discharge. Similarly, antiseptics, perfumed bubble baths or strong soaps can inflame the urethra if you are very sensitive to them. And check to make sure the discharge is actually coming from the urethral opening, rather than from a sore area under the foreskin.

What you should do

Any discharge from the penis needs to be checked out by a doctor – either your doctor or a doctor at a clinic (see page 9). This is because *Chlamydia* and gonorrhea can be easily treated with the correct antibiotics, but can cause problems to you and your future partners if they are not treated properly. Some types of the bacteria that cause gonorrhea are resistant to certain antibiotics, but the clinic will be able to test you to select the correct one.

Inflammation (balanitis)

If the head of your penis (glans) is inflamed – red, sore and itchy – you have balanitis. This is a Greek word meaning 'inflammation of the acorn'. Balanitis usually looks more worrying than it is.

It may simply be a hygiene problem. If you do not wash under the foreskin, a cheesy material, called smegma, accumulates. This can become infected and cause irritation. The solution is to wash carefully with warm water to which you have added enough kitchen salt to make it taste like sea-water.

A milder form of balanitis can appear soon after intercourse, but disappears within about a day. This is caused by allergy to thrush in your partner's vagina. If she is treated the problem will go.

Balanitis can sometimes be caused by a skin disease, such as psoriasis. Psoriasis can occur on the penis without you having it anywhere else. On the glans, it looks red and shiny (unlike on other parts of the body where it is silvery and scaly). In this situation antifungal treatment will not have any effect, but your doctor can prescribe a steroid cream.

Finally, check your soaps and shower gels. Balanitis can sometimes be a sensitivity to perfumes in soaps and detergents. Never put disinfectant in the bath, as this can be very irritating.

Thrush

If your penis is swollen, intensely itchy and very red, you probably have thrush (also known as *Candida*, a yeast). Occasionally this can be the first sign of diabetes, so check with your doctor. It is cured with antifungal cream or tablets.

What to do about balanitis

- Change to a simple, unperfumed soap.
- Put two handfuls of salt in the bath but no other additives (no bubble bath, no bath oils, no disinfectants).
- Don't use 'biological' or 'enzyme' powders when washing your underpants.
- Ask your partner to visit her doctor or a clinic to check for thrush (especially if your balanitis occurs after sex).
- See your doctor – if your balanitis is severe, ask for a diabetes check; if anti-thrush treatment doesn't work, ask your doctor if it could be psoriasis.

Opening in the wrong place

"The opening on my penis isn't at the end, it's just underneath. And my urine sprays about"

Normally, the opening of the urethra (the passage for urine and semen) is at the end of the penis, in the middle of its head (glans). About 1 in every 300 males is born with the opening on the underside, and the middle of the glans just has a blind dimple. This is called *hypospadias*. It tends to run in families; if one child has hypospadias, his brothers have a 1 in 20 chance of also having it.

In 65% of men with hypospadias, the opening is on the underside of the head of the penis, near where it joins the shaft, but it can be anywhere along the underside of the shaft or even at the root of the penis near the testicles. If the opening is on the shaft, the end of the penis may bend when it is erect; this does not occur if the opening is near the head. The foreskin is often abnormal as well; part of it is missing on the underside of the penis, so it looks like a hood.

Hypospadias does not make you incontinent because the urine flow is controlled by the neck of the bladder which is higher up inside the body. However, it can make it difficult to direct the stream of urine accurately, and some men with this condition choose to sit down when they pass urine.

Severe hypospadias, where the opening is on the shaft or near the testicles, will have been noticed at birth, and will have been put right by an operation at the age of 12–18 months. Babies with slight hypospadias, where the opening is on the head of the penis, not far from the dimple, do not always have an operation. If you have hypospadias that was not operated on but which bothers you, because of the appearance of the foreskin or because you cannot control the direction of the urine stream, ask your doctor for a referral to a urological surgeon who will be able to give you more information and discuss the options. Seeing a surgeon does not commit you to having an operation.

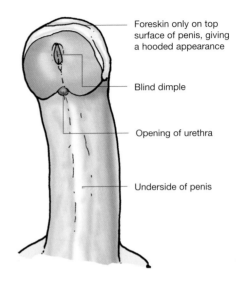

Foreskin only on top surface of penis, giving a hooded appearance

Blind dimple

Opening of urethra

Underside of penis

Hypospadias

Size

Most men can't think rationally about penis size, and they certainly don't have a clear idea of what the average is. According to the Kinsey Institute, many American men think the average erect penis is 25 cm (almost 10 inches) long, and feel worried that they don't measure up. In fact, when researchers at the University of California measured the penises of 80 normal men they found that:

- without an erection (flaccid), the average length was 8.8 cm (just under 3 $\frac{1}{2}$ inches)
- the average flaccid penis could be stretched to 12.4 cm (about 4 $\frac{3}{4}$ inches)
- the average length when erect was 12.9 cm (just over 5 inches).

Of the men studied, many had penises that were larger or smaller than the average. They also found that the length of the penis when flaccid does not predict the size when erect – smaller penises expand more when erect. So, the researchers found the average erect penis to be about 13 cm long, regardless of whether it is 5 cm or 10 cm long when it is flaccid.

A different group of researchers, in Brazil, found the average erect length to be 14.5 cm (5 $\frac{3}{4}$ inches) and the average measurement round the erect penis was 11 cm (just over 4 $\frac{1}{4}$ inches).

Research has also shown that most men don't have a very clear idea of the size of their own penis. Looked at from above, it looks shorter than it really is.

Losing a paunch

If you are carrying a few excess pounds on your abdomen, the first part (called the root) of your penis will be buried in the fat. This makes it look shorter than it really is. Losing weight will make the penis grow!

Penis enlargement

The shaft of the penis can be made thicker by injecting fat from another part of the body (usually the abdomen) under the skin of the penis. The glans (which is the head of the penis) stays the same size, and so it may look a bit out of proportion. The fat tends to be absorbed by the body, so the injections have to be repeated two or three times a year. The fat can sometimes form unsightly nodules, and there can be puckering of the skin and scarring.

The penis can be made longer by a surgical operation in which the ligaments that attach the penis to the pubic bone are cut. This makes the penis hang down further when it is limp, and longer when erect. But, because it no longer has the support of the ligaments, the erect penis will not point as high as before. The operation can be risky, because important nerves that carry sensation can be damaged and infection or bleeding can also occur. If you are considering this operation, make sure that you find a reputable surgeon. This may be difficult, because not many surgeons are willing to do this operation.

A safer approach is to have a suprapubic lipectomy to remove fat from the lower abdomen above the root of the penis. This makes the whole length of the penis more visible.

Tight foreskin

In small children the foreskin is stuck to the glans, but normally begins to separate at about the age of 3. After the age of 7, you should be able to pull your foreskin back over the head (or glans) of your penis. If you cannot do this, it is too tight. This is called *phimosis*. If this is the case, you won't be able to wash under your foreskin properly, so a white, cheesy material called smegma can accumulate. Also, if phimosis is severe it may be painful when the penis is erect.

Some men have phimosis from childhood, but it can also occur late in life, perhaps as a result of several thrush infections affecting the glans. Another common reason is a skin condition called *balanitis xerotica obliterans* which makes the foreskin pale and thickened. The cause of this condition is not known; it is not an infection.

There is no point in trying to force the foreskin back. You will only cause painful cracks on the inside of the foreskin, which will scar as they heal and make it worse. You probably need a circumcision operation, in which the surgeon separates the foreskin from the glans (if it is stuck down), cuts the foreskin away and closes the incision with stitches.

The glans will seem very sensitive after the operation, because it is not used to being exposed. Wear loose boxer shorts and use a condom during sex for the first month or two.

If the doctor thinks the cause is balanitis xerotica obliterans, steroid creams will be used first. This often relieves the condition for several years, but eventually circumcision is usually needed.

Other penis problems: see pages 60, 70, 78, 86, 99, 172.

USEFUL CONTACTS
Impotence Resource Center
Sexual Function Health Council
American Foundation for Urologic Disease
1128 N. Charles Street
Baltimore, Maryland 21201
(800) 433-4215
www.impotence.org

piles (hemorrhoids)

Anal canal

The last 3 cm of the gut is called the anal canal. Its wall is very muscular, and the muscles keep the anus closed (except when feces, or stools, are passed). A network of small veins lies just under the lining of the anal canal. These veins form a soft, spongy pad that acts as an extra seal to keep the canal closed until you go to the lavatory. The lining of the gut is very slimy (so that feces can pass along easily); the extra seal stops the slime (mucus) from leaking out.

What are hemorrhoids?

The small veins that form the extra seal described above can become stretched and bulging – like varicose veins in the leg. If this happens, they are called piles or hemorrhoids. When feces are passed, the pile may be pushed down the anal canal to the outside, and this is called a prolapsed pile.

Doctors classify piles into three types.

- First-degree piles are swollen veins that always remain in their usual position in the anal canal.
- Second-degree piles are pushed down (prolapsed) when feces are passed, but return to their starting position afterwards.
- Third-degree piles are pushed down (prolapsed) when feces are passed, or come down at other times. They do not go back by themselves.

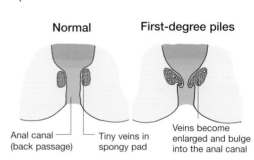

Normal

First-degree piles

Anal canal (back passage)

Tiny veins in spongy pad

Veins become enlarged and bulge into the anal canal

Second- and third-degree piles

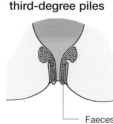

Faeces or straining, can push the piles down

Who gets hemorrhoids?

Most people suffer from hemorrhoids at some time, but usually they are nothing more than a temporary problem. Many experts believe that they are caused by continuous high pressure in the veins, which occurs because humans stand upright. They are particularly common in pregnancy because of the additional pressure from the baby, and because of hormonal changes. Sometimes they result from straining hard to pass feces – which is more likely if you don't eat enough fiber – or to lift a heavy weight. They are *not* caused by sitting on hot radiators or cold, hard surfaces, or by sedentary jobs.

What are the symptoms of hemorrhoids?

The symptoms of hemorrhoids can come and go. There are four main ones:
- itching and irritation
- aching pain and discomfort
- bleeding
- a lump.

Itching and irritation probably occur because the lumpy hemorrhoids stop acting as soft pads to keep the mucus in; instead, a little mucus leaks out and irritates the area round the anus. Pain and discomfort comes from swelling around the pile, and from scratching of the lining of the anal canal by feces as they pass over the lumpy area. The scratching also causes bleeding, which is bright red and may be seen on the feces or on the toilet paper. A pile that has been pushed down (i.e. a second- or third-degree pile) may be felt as a lump at the anus.

How you can help yourself

Most hemorrhoids get better in a few days without any treatment, but there are several ways of relieving the discomfort.
- Wash the area gently with warm, salty water, to get rid of mucus that has leaked out.
- Use soft toilet paper, and dab rather than wipe.
- Don't scratch.
- Avoid constipation by eating lots of fresh fruit and vegetables and bran cereal. Aim for a stool which is soft enough to change its shape as you push it out.
- Drink plenty of fluids.
- If you can feel a lump, try pushing it gently upwards; try to relax your anus as you do so.
- Buy a hemorrhoid cream from a pharmacy, but do not use it for more than a week.

To stop hemorrhoids returning

- Continue the high fiber diet to keep your stools soft.
- Do not put off opening your bowels, take your time over the process, and avoid straining.

When to see your doctor

See your doctor if the symptoms last longer than a week. You should also see your doctor if you have bleeding, to ensure that there is not some other cause. Your doctor will examine your anus, feel inside the anal canal and may also insert a small metal tube an inch or two into the anal canal to give a better view.

Treatments for hemorrhoids

First-degree hemorrhoids usually go away on their own if constipation is avoided, but second- and third-degree piles often need hospital treatment.

Only a few people need an operation; most are treated by photocoagulation, phenol injections or banding. There is usually no need for a general anesthetic or to stay in the hospital overnight.

Photocoagulation uses infrared light to damage the area of the pile. This takes just a few seconds and is painless. As the area heals, it scars. This scarring keeps the blood vessels of the pile in place. Most people have three or four areas that need treatment so have to return several times, at monthly intervals, for more treatments.

Injection of phenol in almond oil is another method of causing scarring in the area.

Banding involves placing a small rubber band at the base of the pile, so that it pinches the lining of the anal canal. This again causes some scarring. It is more effective than the other treatments but has some drawbacks. Some people feel faint and nauseous just after the bands are put on, and they can be quite painful for the following 48 hours.

(Also see page 40 – bottoms)

sex

*"Although I love my partner as much as ever,
I seem to have lost interest in sex"*

- "All this fuss about sleeping together. For physical pleasure I'd sooner go to the dentist any day." (Evelyn Waugh, British writer)
- "I know it does make people happy, but to me it's just like having a cup of tea." (Cynthia Payne, after her acquittal of a charge of controlling prostitutes in a famous case in 1987)
- 37% of men have sex less than once every two weeks (MORI/Esquire poll of 800 men aged 18–45, 1992)

No interest in sex

Sexual appetite *(libido)* tends to wax and wane – there are periods in our lives when we have little desire for sex, and other periods when sex assumes an over-riding importance. Most of the time we are somewhere in between. So losing interest in sex is probably a temporary phase, and not a disaster. In fact it is only a problem if it means there is an imbalance between our desires and those of our partner, if it makes our partner feel unloved and frustrated, or if we ourselves feel unhappy because of it. It is also important to remember that most people are having much less sex than everyone else thinks, as has been shown by many surveys. All the same, there may be a reason for lack of sexual desire which can be remedied.

Reasons in both men and women

Depression is one of the most common reasons. Surveys show that about two out of three people with depression lose interest in sex, as a result of imbalances in brain biochemistry. So it is not something that you should blame yourself for.

Medications, such as antidepressants, tranquilizers and beta-blockers, can damp down sex drive.

Sexual side-effects of antidepressant drugs

Women

- Loss of desire
- Vaginal dryness (so intercourse is uncomfortable)
- Difficulty having an orgasm

Men

- Loss of desire
- Erection problems
- Delayed ejaculation

Stress and physical illnesses take their toll on every aspect of life, including sexuality. It is difficult to be enthusiastic about sex if you are worried, tired, in pain or generally under par.

Relationship problems of any kind can depress libido (although some couples find their sex life improves when other aspects of their relationship are rocky).

Something in the past can affect the present, such as memories of sexual abuse, or a demoralizing sexual relationship.

Reasons in women

A contraceptive method you aren't comfortable with, or worries about infection can trigger a loss of interest in sex. For example, you may have noticed some vaginal discharge, or something about your partner's genitals, and are worrying that you or your partner could have a sexually transmitted disease. Some contraceptive pills, particularly those with a high progesterone content, can reduce sexual desire.

A new baby is very demanding of time and energy, hormone balances are changing and there may be soreness from stitches. So it is not surprising that 50% of women do not have much interest in sex for many months after childbirth (although 1 in 5 women feels more sexual than before). The American sexologists Masters and Johnson found that 47% of women had little desire for sex for at least 3 months after having a baby. Another survey asked women about their sex life 30 weeks after having a baby: only

25% were as sexually active as before, most said their sexual desire was much reduced, and 22% had almost stopped having any sex at all.

Breast-feeding causes temporary vaginal dryness and discomfort (because of the high levels of the breast-feeding hormone, prolactin), making sex seem even less attractive.

Painful intercourse is obviously a turn-off. This can happen because the vagina is dry (see page 181) or for various other reasons (see page 126). In some women the pelvic and nearby muscles clamp up so strongly when intorcourse is attempted that it is uncomfortable, painful or even downright impossible; this is called vaginismus and is discussed on pages 127–128.

Reasons in men
Pressure to perform well in bed seems to be increasing – fuelled by media images of the ever-potent, ever-ready male. A man is expected always to be able to perform sexually. At the same time, modern society expects him to deal with increasing stresses in the workplace, to do his share of household tasks, to be an intellectual companion and emotional support to his partner, and to be a perfect father. It is no wonder that he finds he cannot perform sexually. Over the past decade, the number of couples going to relationship counseling with difficulties blamed on lack of sexual desire in the male partner has doubled.

Heavy drinking is a common cause of loss of interest in sex (and problems with erections). This is because alcohol eventually reduces the production of testosterone by the testes, interferes with processing of testosterone (male hormone) by the cells of the body, and affects the parts of the brain that control hormone balance.

A low testosterone level is seldom the reason for a loss of sex drive, but your doctor can check this quite easily.

Questions to ask yourself
- *Is this really a problem, are my expectations unrealistic, what do I really want, is it affecting my relationship?* You and your partner may feel the situation is quite acceptable. On the other hand, it may be affecting your self-esteem and your relationship.

- *Am I depressed?* Feelings of sadness, hopelessness and helplessness, with lack of energy and disturbed sleep, and an inability to find anything enjoyable are symptoms of depression. Modern antidepressants are very effective at treating depression, and are not addictive. As your depression gradually lifts, your sex life will improve. If this doesn't happen, it may be that the tablets are curing the depression, but their side-effect is making the sex problem worse. Don't stop taking the medication; mention the problem to your doctor, who will be able to change the dose or use a different antidepressant.
- *Am I drinking too much?* If so, try to cut down.
- *Have I started taking any new medications?* A drug is unlikely to be the cause if you had already gone off sex before starting it, but otherwise it is worth checking with your doctor to see if any medication could be responsible.
- *Is there any other physical reason?* If you are tired or physically unwell it is quite reasonable to wish to put your sex life on hold for a while.
- *Is there any specific aspect of our sex life that is putting me off?* A relatively simple problem, such as the type of contraception or pain on intercourse, can be dealt with by a visit to your doctor or family planning clinic. However, there may be a problem which is easy to put your finger on but less easy to deal with. This could be anything – your partner's standards of cleanliness, the type of sexual activities your partner wants, lack of privacy, a suspicion that your partner has a sexually transmitted disease, a triggering of unpleasant memories of sexual abuse. Unfortunately, this type of problem doesn't usually go away on its own, but a counselor (see Useful Contacts) will be able to help you find the best way of dealing with it.
- *Is my loss of interest in sex really because I am unhappy about other aspects of the relationship?* If so, tackle these issues, perhaps with the help of a counselor.

Painful sex

"I hate having sex these days – it's too painful"

There are lots of reasons why sex may become painful – even when the problem has been sorted out it can take a long time before sex becomes enjoyable again. You definitely need help from your doctor for this symptom – it's not something you can sort out on your own.

Before you see your doctor, try to be clear in your mind whether the pain occurs:
- when your partner attempts to put his penis into your vagina (*superficial* pain)
- when the erect penis is fully inserted and during thrusting (*deep* pain)
- in the hours after sex.

Causes of pain at the entrance of the vagina during sex

After childbirth, some women experience pain when they start having sex again. It is more likely after the first baby. Sometimes it is due to an episiotomy that hasn't healed properly. The pain almost always goes away after about 3 months.

A dry vagina is one of the most common reasons – see page 181.

Infections, such as thrush or herpes, make the vulva (lips round the opening of the vagina) sore. Vaginal discharge causes chaffing of the skin, which makes the problem worse.

Blocked Bartholin's glands. Bartholin's glands are just inside the opening of the vagina, one on each side. They help produce lubrication for sex. If the opening of a Bartholin's gland becomes blocked, it swells up into a cyst. Bacteria may enter the cyst, turning it into a painful abscess.

Skin irritants such as perfumed soaps, bubble baths, biological (which means that they contain enzymes) washing powders, 'intimate' deodorants and spermicides can all make the vulva sore.

When sex causes pain deep inside

Pelvic inflammatory disease is an infection of the Fallopian tubes (the tubes, one each side, that carry the egg from the ovaries to the uterus). These tubes lie close to the top of the vagina, so sex causes a deep pain.

Endometriosis is a peculiar condition, in which some of the tissue that normally lines the uterus (sometimes called the womb) lies outside the uterus, in the pelvic cavity. No one knows why it occurs, though it seems to be quite common. Many women have no symptoms from it, but if the tissue is lying behind the uterus it can cause painful sex, especially on deep thrusting. A sign of endometriosis is bad period pains – especially if they last throughout the period.

Pelvic pain syndrome. For two out of every three women with deep pain during sex, no cause can be found; you may have to accept that you have pelvic pain syndrome. This syndrome is not fully understood, but it is related to stress. One possible, but not proven, explanation is that, in some women, chronic stress alters the flow of blood in the veins of the pelvis, so that the pelvis becomes congested. If you are easily aroused during sex, but have difficulty reaching orgasm, the problem becomes worse because the pelvic congestion is not relieved. You may then experience a pain that persists after sex for some hours.

Lack of arousal. Intercourse will be uncomfortable if penetration occurs before you are aroused. This is partly because of lack of lubrication, but also because with sexual arousal the upper part of the vagina balloons open. This helps to lift the womb up and away from the thrusts of the penis. If penetration occurs too early, there may be a pain or discomfort felt deep in the middle of the pelvis with each thrust.

Other causes include irritable bowel syndrome (IBS) and cystitis – the bladder and bowel both lie close to the vagina.

Vagina too tight for sex

"We've never managed to have proper sex
– I think my vagina is too small"

The vagina itself is never too small to accommodate a penis – remember that its walls are stretchy enough to allow a full-sized baby to pass along it. But, it can seem too small for sex if the muscles at its entrance go into a spasm when your partner tries to insert his penis. This is a fairly rare condition called *vaginismus*. Some women with vaginismus can insert a tampon without any problem, but others find that trying to insert anything – a tampon, a finger, a penis – makes the muscles contract.

Very occasionally, the penis cannot be inserted because the hymen (which is the membrane at the entrance to the vagina) is unusually tough, but this is very rare indeed.

How the woman feels

Vaginismus is a very distressing condition. It is very painful if your partner attempts to push his way in, and you may feel wary that he may do this. You may also have feelings of guilt and inadequacy, and fear that your partner may leave you. Some women withdraw from all physical contact – even holding hands – in case it leads to sex.

How the partner feels

Partners are usually confused and worried. Your partner will hate the idea of causing you any pain. He may think that his sexual technique is at fault.

What causes vaginismus?

It is really a deep-rooted phobia of penetration, and perhaps of pregnancy or childbirth. The reason is different for each woman: it can result from some unresolved sexual conflict, from sexual abuse or from a belief that sexual activity is undesirable. You may have had a painful vaginal condition that has left you with a conditioned fear of sex.

Vaginismus shouldn't be confused with frigidity: women with vaginismus are often sexually responsive but can't tolerate penetration.

Treatment

Vaginismus can be helped. Relate, the counseling organization, reports that of 3693 women seen over a 2-year period, 80% improved with therapy.

Psychosexual counselling. The therapy is not at all frightening. You will be taught how to relax your vaginal muscles and eventually to insert a small tampon. In due course you will learn to insert larger tampons. If you have a partner, the therapist will start by telling you not to attempt sex. Instead, you will be encouraged to resume non-genital physical contact in very small steps – such as holding hands, sitting close together or putting an arm round each other. Quite late in the program, you and your partner will be shown how you can insert his penis yourself, as if it were a tampon; he lies on his back and is not allowed to move at this stage. Only at the very end of the therapy program will you be encouraged to have proper sex.

What your doctor can do. To get this psychosexual therapy, it is best to talk to your doctor. Explain that you have a problem with sex, and that this problem means that you have not been able to have sex at all. Your doctor will be able to check that there is no physical problem (such as a tough hymen) and will then arrange for psychosexual

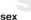
counseling as outlined above. A few doctors are specially trained in this area and will do the therapy themselves. If you do not want your doctor to be involved you can contact a sexual therapist (see Useful Contacts page 136 or look in your phone book for your local branch).

Sex and aging

"We're in our 70s, and our sex life isn't what it was. Are we too old for sex?"

- An American study found that 63% of men and 30% of women aged 80–102 and in good health were enjoying sexual intercourse
- Although studies show that older women are less likely than older men to be sexually active, this is probably only because they are more likely to be alone (women out-live men by 7–8 years on average)

No one is too old for an enjoyable sex life, and many surveys have confirmed that older people continue to enjoy sexual activity into their 80s and 90s. In fact the American Starr-Weiner report showed that sex became more enjoyable with age in about a third of men and an even higher proportion of women. On the other hand, it is undeniable that sex can become problematic as we get older.

Problems for women

For women, the most common physical problem is vaginal dryness, making intercourse uncomfortable. The most common emotional problem is a loss of self-esteem, with a feeling of despair over lost youth and slimness, and a belief that she is no longer sexually attractive. This poor self-image can make her unable to respond to her partner. A woman may also worry that her man is not really up to it, particularly if he has angina or has had a heart attack; she may be secretly terrified that he will die in the attempt.

Problems for men

Men have different problems to contend with as they get older. Some sexual slowing down is natural. For an older man to become aroused, the penis needs to be fondled – sexy thoughts are not enough. Waking with an erection becomes less common. Erections may take longer to develop and be less hard. If the erection is lost before ejaculation, it is less easy to regain. Ejaculation becomes less powerful and more difficult to control. He takes longer to become aroused again after orgasm.

This slowing down is a long way from impotence, but it can make a man panic. At the back of his mind he may have the fear that he is going into a speedy sexual decline and will soon be unable to perform at all. He takes any slight reduction in his body's response – however marginal, and whatever its cause – as the first sign of the onset of impotence. In fact, almost any illness will interfere with sexuality for a while, but the danger is that his 'performance anxiety' takes over, so the fear becomes a self-fulfilling prophecy.

With increasing age, a man is more likely to be taking drugs for high blood pressure (hypertension); many of these drugs cause problems with erections (see page 89). He is also more likely to have conditions such as diabetes which can affect erections and ejaculations.

A man may also have a fixed idea that sex means vigorous, thrusting intercourse with him on top ('missionary position'). As he gets older he finds this more and more difficult, or a heart condition may make him frightened to try. He regards himself as a sexual failure and gives up – instead of experimenting with new positions and new ways of gaining satisfaction.

Problems for men and women

For both men and women, other illnesses can interfere with sexual enjoyment. For example, breathlessness from a chronic chest problem, lack of mobility from arthritis or from a stroke, or simply obesity can make sex difficult. There is also the question of the emotional 'baggage' that the relationship is burdened with; a relationship which has been poor for years may become worse as the older couple find themselves spending more time together.

How you can help yourself

Happiness. Remember that the point of your sex life is to bring greater happiness to you and your partner. If you both feel happy not to continue with your sex life, that's fine. But, if you both wish to have an enjoyable sex life, there is no reason why not.

Expectations. If one partner has needs or expectations not met by the other, sort the problem out rather than let resentment, anger or guilt take over. Counseling (see Useful Contacts) can be very helpful in this situation.

Don't interpret natural sexual 'slowing down' as being near to impotence; try to avoid being too 'performance conscious'.

Poor relationship. If the problem is a poor relationship between you and your partner, get it sorted out (see Useful Contacts). You may feel that your relationship has been unsatisfactory for so many years that it is pointless to try to do anything about it. In fact it is never too late to try to improve things, especially as you and your partner may have many years ahead in which you will be increasingly in each other's company.

Set-backs. If you have a sexual set-back, don't assume it's the beginning of the end of your sex life. It's natural for an illness, or a period of depression, to make you lose the desire for sex, the ability to perform sexually or the ability to respond to your partner. When you are better, your sex life will improve again. If it doesn't, talk to your doctor. For example, you may have been put on some medication that is affecting your sexuality.

If you are worried that sex could damage your heart, or that you or your partner might have a heart attack during sex, talk to your doctor. If you have had a heart attack or heart surgery the hospital should have given you advice about when to resume your sex life.

Sort it out. Don't accept impotence as just a normal part of growing old. If you cannot get an erection that is sufficient for intercourse, discuss it with your doctor, no matter how old you are. There may be a reason that can be put right, and your doctor can explain to you the options to help improve erections (see page 89).

Dry vagina. If a dry vagina is making sex uncomfortable, special lubricants or hormone treatment will help (see page 182), even if it is many years since menopause. Remember that older women need more foreplay to become aroused. Inserting the penis before she is fully lubricated (because the man secretly worries that he will lose his erection) will be uncomfortable or even painful for her.

Try something new! Buy a sex manual and try something new. Sexual experimentation is not just for young people. You will be able to find techniques which you can use for an enjoyable sex life even if you are not physically very fit.

Keep sexually active. Older people who stop sexual activity for a while, perhaps because of separation, bereavement or illness, often have difficulty re-establishing

How aging can affect sex

Good points

- Reduced frequency of sexual desire.
- Likely to have more leisurely lifestyle, with more time for sex.
- Likely to know each other very well, so greater understanding of each other's sexuality.
- Although less frequent, sex may be more enjoyable.

Bad points

- Reduced frequency of sexual desire.
- Arousal takes longer, and needs more genital stimulation.
- Reduced lubrication (women).
- Poor body image (a feeling of being unattractive and undesirable).
- Erections less hard and ejaculations less powerful (men).
- Men are more likely to be taking medication for other medical conditions (for example, high blood pressure) which may affect their erections.
- More likely to have conditions that can affect sexual activity or cause anxiety about having sex.
- Emotional 'baggage'.
- Lack of privacy if not living in own home.
- More difficult to find a new relationship.

sexual function. This is known as *sexual disuse syndrome*. Regular masturbation during such a period of celibacy is healthy and nothing to feel guilty about. It will probably make it easier for you to resume sexual contact in future. Research has also shown that if you are sexually active in your youth and prime you will be more likely to retain your sexual function and interest in old age.

Sex and heart disease

- According to the British Heart Foundation, sex in a long-standing relationship does not put undue stress on the heart, and if you can climb up and down two flights of stairs briskly without symptoms (such as chest pain or breathlessness) you are unlikely to have any problems during sex.
- After a heart attack, you can usually resume sexual activity after 2–3 weeks (but check with your doctor). Start by taking a more passive role, and increase activity gradually.

- If you get chest pain during sex, tell your doctor. He or she will be able to prescribe nitrates for you to keep by the bedside, which should help. If the pain is really troublesome you may need further investigation and treatment.
- If you have a heart condition, don't have sex within 2 hours of a meal or after a hot bath.
- You are very, very unlikely to die during sex with a regular partner. In almost all the cases where this has happened the man was having sex with an unfamiliar partner (like Faure, President of France, who died in 1899 while having sex in a brothel).
- Viagra (sildenafil), a pill for impotence, may not be safe for men with a heart problem. It must not be taken by men who are taking nitrate medication for angina.

Sex during periods

"Is it harmful to have sex during a period?"

- Sex during a period is really a matter of culture (in some cultures menstruation is considered 'unclean') and personal taste.
- Menstrual fluid consists of blood and tissue from the lining of the uterus (womb), with some of the normal 'friendly' bacteria from the vagina. It contains nothing dirty or harmful, so contact with menstrual fluid will not cause irritation of the penis or any other problems.
- Sex at this time will not harm the woman. The menstrual fluid seeps out of the normal small opening in the cervix (see pages 77 and 96). This hole does not become any larger during a period, so there is no need to worry that the penis might poke up into the uterus.

The period is the least fertile time of the woman's cycle, so it is one of the safest times for avoiding pregnancy. However, it is possible to conceive at this time – sperm can live for 3 days, and ovulation could occur earlier than usual, so it might be possible for the sperm to meet up with an egg. To be safe, use contraception.

Remember to remove a tampon beforehand, otherwise it might become pushed up into a corner of the vagina during sex, and then forgotten.

USEFUL CONTACTS

Alcoholics Anonymous (AA)/ www.alcoholics-anonymous.org

Write to:

Grand Central Station

PO Box 459

New York, NY 10163

National Depressive and Manic-Depressive Association

730 N. Franklin Street, Suite 501

Chicago, Illinois   60610-7204 USA

(800) 826-3632

(312) 642-0049

www.ndmda.org

The Endometriosis Association (EA) is a non-profit, self-help organization founded by women for women. The EA is dedicated to providing information and support to women and girls with endometriosis, educating the public as well as the medical community about the disease, and conducting and promoting research related to endometriosis.

Endometriosis Association

International Headquarters

8585 North 76th Place

Milwaukee, WI 53223 USA

(414) 355-2200 /FAX: (414) 355-6065

In North America & Caribbean (800) 992-3636

The Arthritis Foundation has a comprehensive list of local chapters for support on their website at www.arthritis.org.

American Counseling Association
5999 Stevenson Avenue
Alexandria, Virginia 22304-3300
USA
Toll free: 800.347.6647
Tel: 703.823.9800
Fax: 703.823.0252
www.counseling.org

American Association of Marriage and Family Therapy
www.aamft.org
1133 15th Street, NW Suite 300
Washington, DC 20005-2710
Phone: (202) 452-0109
Fax: (202) 223-2329

American Mental Health Counselors Association
801 N. Fairfax Street, Suite 304
Alexandria, VA 22314
800.326.2642 or 703.548.6002
FAX: 703.548.4775
www.amhca.org

American Diabetes Association National Center
1660 Duke Street
Alexandria, VA 22314
(800) 232-3472
www.diabetes.org

National Women's Health Information Center provides access to thousands of publications and organizations with information on hundreds of health topics:

8550 Arlington Blvd.
Fairfax, VA 22031.
1-800-994 WOMAN (1-800-994-9662)
www.4women.gov

shyness – excessive

"I've always been shy, but it's now much worse –
I dread meeting strangers because I know I won't
be able to think of anything to say that isn't boring"

Many people think they are shyer than they actually are. According to psychologists at Stanford University in California, 30–40% of people say they are shy, but when their behavior is observed only 15–20% behave in a shy manner (but of course they may still be feeling shy inside).

An extreme form of shyness, known as social phobia, affects 1–2% of men and 2–3% of women. A phobia is a fear, and people with social phobia have a fear of being the center of attention. They worry that everyone is looking at them and judging them and that they will make a fool of themselves. They fear being introduced to other people. At a party, they will hover round the edge of the room or stay in the kitchen, avoiding being involved and maybe convincing themselves that they are just claustrophobic. It is not that they prefer to be alone – in fact, they want to connect with others – but intense self-consciousness makes this impossible for them. Eating and drinking in public may be very stressful. Some people with social phobia can interact with new people on a one-to-one basis, but go into a total panic if they have to speak or perform in front of a number of people. They may drink too much, in an attempt to give themselves extra confidence.

Treatments for shyness
These are increasingly available, especially for social phobia. The first step is to recognize that your shyness is a real disability that needs help. You then need to explain to your doctor that it is affecting your life, and that you think it is beyond ordinary shyness. The very fact that you have social phobia will make it difficult for you to ask for help. One way round this difficulty is to take with you some information about social phobia (see Useful Contacts) and say to your doctor "I've been reading this, and I think I have this problem." Alternatively, you could write a letter to your doctor beforehand, to prepare the ground.

Cognitive therapy for social phobia

A person with social phobia has very negative thoughts, such as:

- "If the conversation stops, it will be my fault"
- "I won't be able to think of anything to say"
- "I'm boring"
- "I'm a social failure"

Cognitive therapy teaches the person to test out and then to correct these thoughts. For example:

- Deliberately pause during a conversation and see what happens
- Look for real signs (rather than imaginary ones) of whether the other person actually is bored.
- Recognize that a conversation may dry up because the other person has nothing to say. In general, concentrate on past successes rather than failures.

There are various different treatments. Social skills training, in which the individual is taught simple social skills such as how to start a conversation, is one possibility. Another approach is cognitive therapy, in which the individual is taught to think of the social situation in a new way, instead of focusing on their own inadequacies.

In the past, tranquilizing drugs, such as valium, were given to people who were over-anxious in social situations. In fact, they do not really help, and are also addictive. Nowadays, two main groups of drugs are used for social phobia.

- Reversible inhibitors of monoamine oxidase, or RIMAs for short, make the person feel generally more able to participate socially.
- Selective serotonin reuptake inhibitors, or SSRIs for short, help to ease the anxiety symptoms and panic feelings that go with social phobia.

USEFUL CONTACTS

Anxiety, Phobias, and Panic : A Step-By-Step Program for Regaining Control of Your Life (Warner Books) by Reneau Z. Peurifoy is available at your local bookstore on online.

Anxiety & Phobia Workbook by Edmund J. Bourne (Fine Communications) is a self-help workbook for those who suffer from panic attacks or shyness.

American Counseling Association
5999 Stevenson Avenue
Alexandria, Virginia 22304-3300
USA
Toll free: 800.347.6647
Tel: 703.823.9800
Fax: 703.823.0252
www.counseling.org

American Mental Health Counselors Association
801 N. Fairfax Street, Suite 304
Alexandria, VA 22314
800.326.2642 or 703.548.6002
FAX: 703.548.4775
www.amhca.org

skin

"My skin is beginning to look old and wrinkly, and I'm beginning to get some liver spots on my hands"

- In the US alone, people spend $850 million a year on anti-aging skin products
- The French call brown age spots 'les medallions de cimetière' (cemetery medals)
- Cleopatra used red wine – now known to contain AHAs (see below) – on her face
- The Ebers papyrus – an ancient Egyptian papyrus from 1550 BC – has a recipe to cure wrinkles, made from pistachio nuts, wax, poppy seed oil and grass

Aging

Old skin is wrinkled, dry, saggy and has a mottled color. In fact, these changes are more to do with exposure to sunlight than with simply getting old. This is why the exposed areas – hands, face and neck – seem to age faster and look less attractive than the smooth and even skin on, for example, the tummy.

The sun isn't good for skin. It makes it thinner and damages some of its important proteins – collagen, which acts as scaffolding to give skin its strength, and elastin which gives skin its bounce. Even young complexions develop fine wrinkles after sunbathing, giving the skin a coarse, grainy appearance. Collagen also supports the tiny blood vessels in the skin; weakening of the collagen means they show up as broken thread veins ('farmer's face') and bleed more easily. These tiny bruises end up as mottled discoloration. Brownish patches, known as liver spots, gradually develop on sun-exposed areas such as hands and sides of the forehead.

What can be done

Staying out of the sun as much as possible, and using sunscreens, will prevent further damage and may also help the skin improve – there is evidence that the skin can repair itself to some extent, if given half a chance.

Most of the damage is done by UVB light (although UVA is damaging to some extent), so check that your sunscreen filters out UVB as well as UVA. Ideally, you should apply a sunscreen every day, not just on vacation or on sunny days, because even quite low but repeated doses of UVA and UVB can wreak havoc with collagen and elastin. Unfortunately there is no such thing as a safe tan – a tan is a sign that the skin has already had too much light and is desperately trying to protect itself against further damage. Use fake tans and sunscreen instead.

Moisturizers cannot prevent or really get rid of wrinkles. They coat the skin with a very thin layer of oil or silicone, which prevents it drying out. If skin is dry, wrinkles are more noticeable, so by keeping the skin moist and plump they help to blank out smaller wrinkles. It is best to apply a moisturizer after washing in the morning, while your skin is slightly damp.

Do anti-aging creams work? The Consumers' Association magazine *Which?* selected 12 ordinary moisturizers and 12 anti-aging creams. Four women tested each product, according to the manufacturers' instructions, for 4 weeks. None of the 96 women knew what product they were using. At the end of the trial, they were asked to guess whether they had been using an ordinary moisturizer or an anti-aging cream. Most of the women didn't notice any difference in the look or feel of their skin. Ten of the 48 women using anti-aging creams reported an improvement, but even more of those who had used moisturizers – 18 out of 48 – noticed the same thing. Three-quarters of all the women thought that they had been using a simple moisturizer. *Which?* concluded that 'some of the claims made for the ingredients of anti-aging creams can be substantiated but, in the low concentrations used in the creams, they are unlikely to do more than moisturize your skin.'

Hormone replacement therapy doesn't improve wrinkles, but it makes the skin thicker and less dry and flaky.

Retinoids, such as tretinoin and isotretinoin, are chemicals that are related to vitamin A. They make the skin produce new cells more quickly, so it becomes thicker and more compact. The skin also produces more collagen but less pigment (melanin). After a month or two of use, the skin becomes smoother, fine wrinkles are repaired, age spots fade and the skin color becomes more even, but it doesn't produce totally wrinkle-free skin. If you carry on using the cream, the skin continues to improve for a

How effective is tretinoin cream?

In a study of 251 people with sun-damaged skin aged 29–50, tretinoin cream used once a day for 6 months:

- produced some type of improvement in 79% (however, 48% of people who used only sunscreen and moisturizers also showed improvement)
- made the skin 29.3% less rough
- faded age spots by 37%
- improved wrinkles by 27.1% (measured by taking silicone impressions of the skin)

From *Archives of Dermatology* 1991;127(5):659–65

Verdict: in spite of the hype, tretinoin will not change your skin radically, but it may produce some improvement

few more months, but after 6 months of use there is no further change. If you stop using it, the skin gradually goes back to how it was before. Retinoids do not have any effect on very noticeable wrinkles, such as the deep lines that appear between the nose and mouth, or on thread veins.

To obtain tretinoin you need a doctor's prescription. For the first 2 weeks you apply it every other night; for the next few weeks you apply it every night; after a few weeks, 2 or 3 nights a week is enough. If there is no improvement after 6 months, there is no point in continuing.

Retinoids do irritate the skin, so that there may be dryness and flakiness, sometimes with itching, soreness, redness and a tight feeling. You have to avoid the sun. Some specialists think that retinoids work simply because they irritate the skin, and that the normal skin repair processes then smooth out wrinkles. Other specialists worry that retinoids could increase the risk of skin cancer.

Alpha hydroxy acids or AHAs are chemicals found in fruit juices (hence their name 'fruit acids'), wine, sugar cane and milk, and may be the magic ingredient of old skin recipes containing milk, lemons or wine. They make the skin look better by speeding up the shedding of old, dead cells from the surface of the skin. AHAs have very little effect on wrinkles, though some researchers claim that they also make the skin thicker, help it to hold moisture and improve the elastin.

AHAs are now included in many face creams. When buying, check their concentration. Anything less than 5% won't have much effect, so look for creams containing between 5% and 15%. For the first few weeks they may make the skin flaky.

Stopping smoking is a must – cigarettes cause wrinkling.

Collagen injections into the skin fill in hollows and can help smooth out lines, including deep wrinkles such as nose-to-mouth grooves and frown lines. The collagen is absorbed by the body, so the effect doesn't last and the treatment has to be repeated every 3 to 6 months. It can be painful, and can cause bruising; there is often some redness and swelling on the day of the injection, which fades by the following day. Some people develop hard, red, blotches as a result of an allergic reaction. Collagen injections are available at some private clinics: make sure you choose a reputable one.

Chemical peeling with AHAs, phenol or trichloracetic acid is another treatment given at some private clinics, though it is now being replaced by laser 'resurfacing'. Chemical peeling works by producing a chemical burn on the surface of the skin. As the skin heals, some of the smaller wrinkles and irregularities are smoothed out and there is some improvement in the appearance.

Laser resurfacing of the skin is becoming more common, and the technology is developing fast. The laser removes the outer layer of the skin, called the epidermis, which regrows in 3–6 weeks from the remnants left in the hair follicles and sweat glands (see page 21). During this time, you will look as if you have severe sunburn, as your skin will be red and there may be some weeping. The repair process alters the skin collagen, 'lifting' mini-wrinkles from the skin during the subsequent 4 months. Afterwards, you must always use sunscreen to protect your skin.

Because these skin techniques are so new, discoveries are still being made about the best methods, and what they can and cannot do, and their long-term effects. As with all cosmetic operations and procedures, try to choose a reputable clinic and a well-known doctor; your doctor may be able to advise you. Ask to see 'before and after' photos, and check that the procedures were carried out by the person you are talking to, and are not simply promotional material supplied by the laser manufacturer.

Plastic surgery was the only option before retinoids. It can produce a big improvement in lines at the sides of the eyes and sagging skin of the neck (which retinoids won't help), but will not improve the overall texture of the skin. As with all plastic surgery, make sure you choose a reputable clinic. Ask to see 'before and after' photos, and check that the doctor you are talking to actually did the work shown.

USEFUL CONTACTS

Skin Healthy: Everyone's Guide to Great Skin is a book by Norman Levine (Taylor Publishing Company: ISBN 0-87833-900-0). Written by a dermatologist, this gives you all the facts you need to know about caring for your skin.

snoring

"I've been told I snore. What can I do about it?"

- 24% of men and 14% of women say they know they snore (San Marino survey)
- 71% of wives say their husbands snore, while 51% of husbands say their wives snore (Toronto survey)
- 20% of men in their early 30s snore, but only 5% of women in that age group do
- Snoring is said to have been useful to primitive man, frightening away beasts of prey at night
- Churchill and Mussolini were both famous snorers

What causes snoring?

When we are awake, the muscles of the throat hold the throat open, so that air passes in smoothly as we breathe. During sleep, these muscles relax and the throat sags inwards, causing air turbulence, particularly as we breathe in. Snoring occurs when the roof of the mouth (soft palate and uvula – the uvula is the piece of tissue that dangles at the back of the throat), and sometimes the base of the tongue as well, starts to vibrate intermittently as a result of excessive turbulence. This is particularly likely to happen if you:

- have a small jaw and narrow throat and/or a large uvula and base of tongue
- drink alcohol or take sleeping pills. These make the throat muscles very relaxed, and so worsen turbulence in the throat
- are overweight, particularly if you have a fat neck. This is because more muscle power is needed to hold the throat open if the neck is fat, and so during sleep there will be a greater degree of narrowing of the throat as the muscles relax
- breathe through your mouth rather than your nose; this is because when you breathe through your mouth the air hits the back of the throat head-on, increasing turbulence, whereas in nose breathing it enters the throat parallel with it
- smoke. The reason may be that smoking causes swelling and inflammation of the lining of the throat

145

How snoring occurs

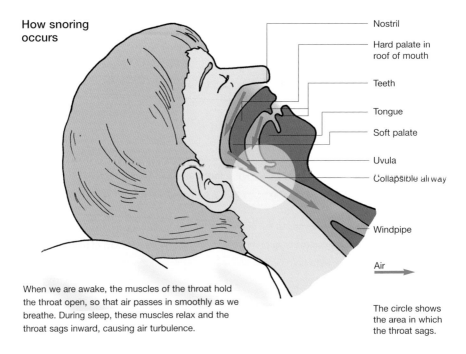

Nostril

Hard palate in roof of mouth

Teeth

Tongue

Soft palate

Uvula

Collapsible airway

Windpipe

Air

When we are awake, the muscles of the throat hold the throat open, so that air passes in smoothly as we breathe. During sleep, these muscles relax and the throat sags inward, causing air turbulence.

The circle shows the area in which the throat sags.

- sleep on your back. When the muscles are relaxed, the throat is particularly narrow in this position
- eat a large meal before bed – a full stomach presses upwards on the diaphragm and can lead to labored breathing.

Is snoring dangerous?

Snoring is not a disease. In fact, it is so common that one could argue that it is almost normal. However, loud snoring may be a sign that the relaxed throat muscles are allowing the throat to become excessively narrow during sleep, and not enough air is getting through with each breath. Sometimes breathing stops altogether for 10 seconds or more, until the body's arousal system causes it to resume; this is called *sleep apnea syndrome*. It is nine times more common in men than women, particularly the overweight, and most sufferers are loud snorers. Men with a collar size of 43 cm (17 inches) have a 30% chance of sleep apnea syndrome.

In sleep apnea you may quickly wake up with a feeling of choking or shortness of breath, or you may hardly wake at all, just enough for the throat muscles to tone up and pull the throat open again. This can happen hundreds of times a night without you being aware of it. Not surprisingly, you will feel tired during the day because of the disturbed sleep and may be aware that sleep is not a refreshing experience. Your bed partner may notice that you are very restless during sleep or that you seem to stop breathing for a few moments, with resumption of breathing signalled by sudden loud snoring.

To see if you are excessively sleepy in the day, check your score on the Epworth Sleepiness Scale. A total score of more than 12 is abnormal.

If you think sleep apnea syndrome is a possibility, consult your doctor, who may refer you to a laboratory that has equipment for assessing disordered breathing during sleep.

Epworth Sleepiness Scale

For each situation:

   Score 0 if you would never doze off
   Score 1 for a slight chance of dozing
   Score 2 for a moderate chance of dozing
   Score 3 for a high chance of dozing

Situation	**Chance of dozing score**
● Sitting reading	....
● Watching TV	....
● Sitting (inactive) in a public place (for example, at the theatre, at a meeting)	....
● As a passenger in a car for an hour	....
● Lying down to rest in the afternoon if circumstances would permit	....
● Sitting talking to someone	....
● Sitting quietly after lunch (no alcohol)	....
● In a car, while stopped for a few minutes in traffic	....

How to stop snoring

There is no shortage of 'cures' for snoring (over 300 anti-snoring devices have been registered at the US patent office alone), but in many cases 'self-help' is effective.

● Lose weight if you are overweight.

● Avoid alcohol, tranquilizers and sleeping pills within 4 hours of bedtime.

- Put a walnut, cork or even a tennis ball into a sock and pin it to the back of your pajamas (use a safety pin). This will encourage you to sleep sideways rather than on your back.
- Tilt the head of your bed up 10 cm (4 inches) by putting bricks under the legs to lessen the effect of gravity on the throat muscles. Alternatively, put a wedge of foam under the bottom sheet at the pillow end. It should be about 75 cm (30 inches) long, 65 cm (26 inches) wide and 20 cm (8 inches) high. Don't use a thick pillow: this will kink your neck and make the problem worse.
- Try sleeping in a whiplash foam collar, to stop the neck kinking.
- Have a coffee or cola drink at night, so your partner gets to sleep first.
- Nostril dilators such as Nozovents, Snoreless and Breathe Right strips can be bought. These encourage nasal breathing and help to prevent mouth breathing. Nozovents have the disadvantage that they lose their springiness after a few weeks and tend to fall out; the Snoreless model has prongs to prevent this. Breathe Right strips (used by some sports players) are self-adhesive strips that you apply to the outside of the nose; they widen the nostrils from the outside.
- Plastic mouth devices (technically called *mandibular advancement splints*) are available to hold the jaw slightly forward while you sleep; when the jaw is in this forward position the airway opens wider. For example, with the Snore Guard, you mold it to fit yourself by placing it in hot water. These devices may be difficult to get used to, but are said to help 70% of snorers.

What your doctor can do

Consult your doctor if you have tried these approaches without success. You should also see your doctor if nostril dilators have relieved the problem; this could mean that you have nasal obstruction that could be dealt with by surgery. You should also see your doctor if you have any of the symptoms of sleep apnea.

In the 1980s, an *uvulopalatopharyngoplasty* operation was a common treatment for people who could not lead normal lives because of their snoring. In this procedure, a 1 cm strip is removed from along the entire free edge of the soft palate, including the uvula. As it heals, it scars, and this stiffens the palate so that it cannot vibrate. The disadvantages are that it is very painful, it will not cure the problem if the base of the tongue vibrates as well as the palate, the voice may change (especially noticed in singers) and cure may not be permanent. After the operation, 5–10% of people find that fluid goes up into the nose when they drink. A more recent technique uses a laser to burn away part of the uvula and soft palate and produce the desired scarring. This technique (*laser palatoplasty*) has fewer side-effects; there will be pain and discomfort in the throat for about 2 weeks afterwards, and some people have a slight feeling of dryness in the throat for several months. These operations improve snoring in about 85% of cases, but the cure is not always permanent, so the long-term success rate is about 66%. A similar technique uses a fine heated needle (*diathermy palatoplasty*).

The other approach is *nasal CPAP,* which stands for nasal continuous positive airways pressure. This involves wearing a mask at night, attached to a machine that delivers air under pressure to keep the throat open. Some people cannot get used to the noise of the machine, or the claustrophobic feeling of wearing a mask.

What your dentist can do

It is possible to have a mandibular advancement splint made-to-measure. These are expensive – costing several hundred dollars. A few dentists have been trained to fit them. If your dentist has not had this training, he or she can refer you to a specialist orthodontist.

USEFUL CONTACTS

American Sleep Apnea Association
1424 K Street NW, Suite 302
Washington, DC 20005
202/293-3650   fax: 202/293-3656
asaa@sleepapnea.org
www.sleepapnea.org

stuttering

"What can I do about my stutter?"

- More men than women stutter
- There is a 20% greater chance of you stuttering if a close relative has a stutter
- There is no difference between stammering and stuttering; they are two words with the same meaning
- People who stutter can usually whisper and sing without stuttering
- Famous stutterers include Moses, Aristotle, Aesop, Virgil, Charles I, Charles Darwin and Somerset Maugham

You should get the help of a speech and language therapist, preferably one who specializes in the treatment of stammering. Your doctor can refer you, or you can get in touch with a therapist yourself (see Useful Contacts). The therapy may be on an individual basis, or may be in a group. If you have already had speech therapy and feel that you were not helped, try again because therapy may have changed and you may have changed.

There is some evidence that stutterers tend to use the right sides of their brains for speech. This is different from most people, who typically use their left side. Maybe there is a grain of truth in the old wives' tale that getting a child to switch from being left-handed to right-handed can cause stuttering.

How to help yourself

There are various ways in which you can help yourself. The British Stammering Association suggests the following approach.

Defining the problem

What do you actually do when you stutter?

- Do you repeat sounds (s..s..s..supper) or syllables (su..su..su..supper)?
- Do you prolong sounds (sssssssupper)?
- Do you get blocked in speech so that you are unable to make any sound (s..upper)?

- Do you close your eyes or rush through speech?
- Do you try to avoid the word by changing it for another that is easier to say?
- Do you give up speaking altogether?

You also need to consider what you feel about your stutter.

- Do you think it is severe or quite mild?
- Do you think it is holding you back in your social life or at work?
- Is it better in some situations and with some people?
- How do you feel when you stutter: embarrassed? annoyed? frustrated?
- Do you get angry at other people, at yourself, or both?

Tackling the problem piece by piece. Having analyzed your stutter, tackle it one element at a time, starting with something you feel you might be able to change. For example, you might take one sentence of your speech two or three times a day and make a special effort to say that sentence slowly and calmly. Do not allow yourself to rush or panic; when speaking more slowly, most people stutter less. Or perhaps you might try to concentrate on not looking away from people, or not closing your eyes when you stutter.

Don't try to hide your stutter. You have probably adopted some 'avoidance behaviors' to hide or avoid your stutter. The problem is that the more you avoid, the more you need to go on avoiding. If you are avoiding very successfully, you may be thought to be fluent by workmates, partner and friends, but you have to be constantly vigilant to maintain this fluency. Your stutter does not improve or go away because you hide it.

Try to reduce the number of times that you avoid saying a word, talking to a particular person or speaking in a certain situation. As well as experimenting with stuttering more openly, you may find it useful to try to talk about your stutter to one or two people who are close to you. You will start to learn that people are not as critical as you thought.

Degrees of fluency. You may think there are only two possibilities – either you stutter or you are fluent. Watch and listen carefully when people are speaking on buses, on radio phone-ins, at home and in shops. Is everyone as fluent, concise and articulate as you imagined? You may discover that many apparently fluent speakers are, in fact, quite hesitant when speaking, and that there is not such a clear division between speaking fluently and stammering. You may then begin to accept that you do not have to be fluent all the time.

Helping a stutterer

- Don't give unhelpful advice, such as 'slow down' or 'take a deep breath'. Just accept that the person stutters.
- Do be patient and maintain eye contact with the stutterer when he or she speaks.
- Don't interrupt or finish words or sentences for the stutterer.
- Concentrate on what is being said, rather than how it is being said.

USEFUL CONTACTS

National Stuttering Association
www.nsastutter.org
nsastutter@aol.com

Phone the toll-free national hotline at 1-800-364-1677 or send them a FAX at (714) 693-7554 for information about local chapters and support groups.

stretch marks

*"I'm sick of my stretch marks.
Can anything be done about them?"*

What are they?

Stretch marks look like thin, stretched tissue, and that is more or less what they are. They appear in people who put on or lose weight rapidly. The upper layer of the skin is normal, but in the lower layer, the collagen and elastin which give the skin its strength and elasticity have become thinner and broken. At first, the marks look reddish-purple. This is because the stretched skin is more transparent and the small blood vessels that lie deep in the skin, show through. Later, the blood vessels contract. The purplish colour then fades to white, which is just the fat under the skin showing through.

Who gets them?

Stretch marks often appear on the breast and abdomen during pregnancy. The reason is partly hormonal. During pregnancy, hormones have the job of softening the collagen ligaments of the pelvis, so that the tissues can stretch easily during childbirth. Unfortunately, the skin collagen softens as well, allowing stretch marks to form easily.

Bodybuilders and yo-yo dieters can also get them on the upper arms, chest and thighs. Growing adolescents can get them on their backs, looking like a series of horizontal lines.

Preventing stretch marks

- Try to avoid yo-yo dieting. If you are overweight, aim to lose it slowly (don't aim to lose more than a pound a week).
- If you are pregnant there is not much you can do, except keep your fingers crossed and think "this is a small price to pay for a beautiful baby!" Rubbing baby oil into the abdomen each night might help. Various special creams and oils are promoted for preventing stretch marks, but there is no proof that they are effective.

Curing stretch marks

Stretch marks are permanent in the sense that the skin in these areas will never be completely normal. However, after a time they contract down into much less obvious, thin, whitish scars.

Some creams contain collagen, and claim that they will improve stretch marks. There is no evidence that they do so. In fact, collagen and elastin put onto the surface of the skin can't penetrate into the deeper layers.

At an early stage, when they are still red, stretch marks can be treated by laser. The red blood cells in the small blood vessels absorb the energy from the laser beam and convert it into heat, which then seals the blood vessels. This gets rid of the red colour and might speed up the contracting process, but is uncertain whether it will make any difference in the long run. It costs several hundred dollars, and may not be covered under insurance. As with any cosmetic treatment, check that the clinic is reputable; your doctor can probably advise you.

Recently, doctors in New York have been treating old, white stretch marks with lasers. They claim this improves the stretch marks, but they don't know why it does! They think the treatment may possibly boost the production of new collagen in the skin.

Another approach to the treatment of early stretch marks is tretinoin (see page 141); doctors at the University of Michigan claim that this produces some improvement in 80% of users, but other researchers have not found any effect.

sweaty armpits

*"I have to keep my arms close into my body, because
I know there will be underarm sweat stains on my shirt"*

- Victorians sponged their armpits with sulphuric acid
- In the 1950s, you could be sedated with barbiturates or recommended for a course of X-ray treatment to help with this embarrassing problem

Sweat is not smelly in itself, but it quickly becomes a breeding ground for bacteria. These bacteria break it down to produce fatty acids. It is these fatty acids which have the acrid, penetrating, pungent 'stale sweat' smell. So the problem can be approached in two ways – sweating itself can be prevented, or the bacteria that cause the smell can be attacked.

How to help yourself
Commercial antiperspirants – you have probably tried most commercial deodorants and antiperspirants, but check the labels and look for one with a different active ingredient.

Shave your armpits – hair holds sweat and gives the bacteria more to work on.

Chlorhexidine 0.05% solution is an antibacterial liquid that you can buy from the pharmacy. Apply it daily. It won't prevent sweating, but will kill the bacteria.

20% aluminum chloride is the next thing to try if chlorhexidine hasn't done the trick. It can be bought from the pharmacist (ask for Drichlor or Anhydrol Forte). Use it as follows.
- Before going to bed, wash and dry your armpits thoroughly. If you apply the solution to wet skin, a chemical reaction takes place that produces hydrochloric acid, which can irritate skin and tarnish jewelery.

- Apply the solution when you are lying down in bed. This sounds odd, but armpit sweating switches off when you lie flat, and the solution will be more effective if applied then. The solution works by passing into the openings of the sweat glands, causing them to swell up and block, but if sweat is pouring out of the glands when you apply the solution, it won't be able to get in.
- Don't apply it directly after shaving, or the skin may become sore.
- Wash off the solution in the morning, and don't reapply until bedtime.
- If it proves effective reduce the application to every other night, and then to once or twice a week.

Surgical removal of some skin from the armpit is an option if aluminium chloride doesn't work. It can be dramatically effective. Under a local anesthetic, the surgeon removes a section of skin about 4 cm x 1.5 cm, taking away the most troublesome sweat glands. A new technique is removal of the sweat glands by sucking them out of the deep layer of the skin (liposuction method).

A sympathectomy operation to cut the sympathetic nerves that control sweating is a last resort. Some surgeons are now able to do a sympathectomy using keyhole surgery. A general anesthetic is required. The sympathetic nerves lie in the chest just under the second, third and fourth ribs on each side. The surgeon operates through an incision in the chest wall and destroys the nerves using an electrical current. After the operation, you can return to a sedentary job after 1–2 weeks, and to a manual job after 2–3 weeks. The success rate is 30–40%. The main drawback is that the body may compensate by increasing sweating elsewhere – usually the trunk, but sometimes the feet – so you may end up swapping sweaty armpits for a sweaty abdomen. This happens in between a third and three-quarters of people who have had the operation. In 1 in 100, this 'compensatory' sweating is very severe, and they regret they had the operation. Unfortunately, the operation cannot be reversed.

sweaty feet

"My feet smell so bad that I dread buying shoes, and I sometimes buy them without trying them on first"

- Each person has 3–4 million sweat glands
- At rest, a normal person loses about half a liter of sweat a day
- The sweat glands are capable of producing 12 liters of sweat in 24 hours
- Humans rely on the evaporation of sweat to protect the body against a hot environment – most other animals rely on insulation or panting

Sweat is not smelly in itself, but bacteria quickly work on it to produce fatty acids. It's these that have the acrid, penetrating, pungent 'stale sweat' smell. So the problem can be approached in two ways. Either the sweating itself can be prevented, or the bacteria that cause the smell can be attacked.

One of the main causes of sweaty, smelly feet is wearing the wrong socks or footwear. Shoes with plastic or other synthetic fabric linings don't allow even normal amounts of sweat to evaporate and don't absorb it either, so the foot stays wet. Synthetic socks have the same effect, especially if they're tight.

What to do

- Throw out all your nylon socks. Replace them with socks that are 60–70% wool combined with 40–30% man-made fiber. Socks that are all cotton are not as good because they don't hold as much moisture without becoming sodden, and all-wool socks become clammy. Make sure your socks have a close weave and are not too tight. If necessary, wear a second pair of the correct socks over the first pair to increase absorbency. Wear clean socks every day. Wash socks on the hottest cycle. After washing, rinse your socks in antiseptic, diluted 20 times, and let them dry naturally.
- Look for socks that have been treated with chemicals that kill the bacteria that produce the smell. This technology was first developed in Japan.

- Check the linings of your shoes. Leather shoes often have a plastic lining, so be sure to choose all-leather shoes without a lining or ones that are lined with leather.
- Avoid wearing sneakers for long periods. Most sneakers are insulating and synthetic – ideal conditions for cheesy feet.
- Check the soles of your feet for hard skin. Hard skin is dead skin, and it becomes soggy when damp, providing an ideal environment for bacteria. Remove it with a pumice stone.
- Bathe your feet in warm water with a few drops of tea-tree oil added. Tea-tree oil has antibacterial properties. Dry your feet thoroughly.
- Check between your toes for fungal infections such as athlete's foot. Fungal infections are another cause of smelly feet. Fungi also thrive when the feet are warm and moist. The skin between the toes will look red and soggy. Buy an antifungal foot spray, which is more effective than the antifungal foot powders. Keep using the spray for 10 days after the symptoms have gone. If the problem persists, see your doctor.

Try using

20% aluminium chloride (see page 155). It is available from your chemist. Before applying it, take great care to dry the feet properly. If your feet are the least bit damp, the aluminium chloride won't work.

Potassium permanganate soaks (1 in 10 000 aqueous solution) if smell is the main problem. Your local pharmacy will be able to order potassium permanganate for you. Soak your feet twice a day for 10 minutes. This helps to kill the bacteria and may reduce the sweating. Soaking can irritate some people's skin, so stop the treatment if this starts to occur.

If it gets serious

Iontophoresis is a treatment available through some hospital physiotherapy departments. It is a way of applying an anticholinergic drug directly into the skin of the foot. Anticholinergic drugs block the action of the nerves responsible for sweating. The treatment involves the passing of an electrical current through a solution of the drug into the skin. It is painless and effective, but is tedious. At first, treatment is weekly but it is gradually decreased to once every 3 or 4 weeks. Some practitioners claim that iontophoresis works just as well with water as with a solution of a drug.

Anticholinergic drugs, such as propantheline bromide, can be prescribed by your doctor. As these block the action of the nerves responsible for sweating, they are fairly effective. However, their side-effects – drying of the mouth, blurring of vision, constipation, sedation – are probably worse than the sweating!

A surgical procedure, called lumbar sympathectomy, is a last resort if the sweating is really disabling. It involves destroying the nerves that control foot sweating but, like any operation, it has risks.

sweaty hands

"I try to avoid shaking hands – mine are always so sweaty"

You can disguise sweaty hands to some extent by smoothing back your hair – so that you wipe your hands on your hair – before you shake hands with anyone. But it can be embarrassing if you leave sweaty handprints on anything you touch.

What you can do

First ask yourself whether your sweaty hands mean that you are excessively anxious in certain situations. If this is the case, dealing with the anxiety will lessen the problem (see page 138).

You may not be excessively anxious – it may simply be that even slight, normal anxiety triggers your hands to sweat excessively. If this is the case, you can try rubbing your palms with astringent oils, such as cypress or geranium (from health stores). Alternatively, try 20% aluminium chloride, painting it onto your hands as described for armpits on page 155. You can buy aluminium chloride from chemists without a prescription. Unfortunately, it is not as effective for hands as for armpits.

If this doesn't work you need to see your doctor.

What your doctor can do

If the sweating is particularly associated with anxiety and stress, your doctor may prescribe beta-blocker tablets. Alternatively he or she can refer you to a hospital physiotherapy department for iontophoresis treatment (see page 158).

For a permanent cure you could consider a sympathectomy operation (see page 156). This is often done to control excessive sweating under the arms, but it is 95% successful for sweating of the hands. The result is immediate; you wake from the anesthetic with dry, warm hands.

swollen testicles

*"One of my balls is swollen –
I think it must be cancer"*

It is a good idea to examine your testicles regularly, so that you become familiar with your own anatomy. Then you will be able to notice if anything unusual develops.

- The testicles make sperm. They are oval in shape, and are usually about 4–5 cm long, 3 cm wide and 2 cm thick. One is often slightly larger than the other.
- The epididymis is a sausage-shaped lump stuck onto the back and top of each testicle. It is actually a coil of tiny tubes, which carry and store the sperm. If uncoiled, they would be about 15–20 feet long.
- The spermatic cords lead upwards from behind the epididymis. They carry the sperm towards the penis, and also contain blood vessels.
- The scrotum is the skin sac that contains the testicles and the epididymis.

The testicle

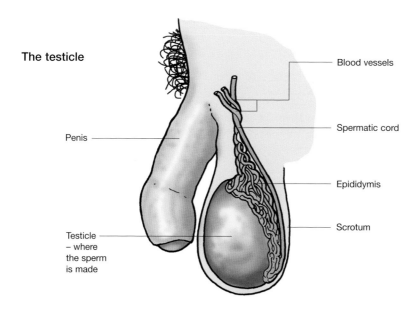

Blood vessels

Spermatic cord

Penis

Epididymis

Scrotum

Testicle
– where
the sperm
is made

Cancer is a possibility with any lump in the scrotum, and it is important to detect it early because the cure rate is now over 90%. However, most swellings in the scrotum turn out to be non-cancerous. For example, it is common to have small lumps and cysts in the epididymis and in the spermatic cord. Another common occurrence is for the veins in the cord to become lumpy and twisted, and feel like a 'bag of worms'.

It is important that all lumps in the scrotum are examined by a doctor, so even if you think the swelling is not cancerous have it checked anyway. If your doctor is not sure, he will arrange for you to have an ultrasound scan, which is painless.

How to examine your testicles

- The best time is after a warm bath or shower, when the skin of the scrotum is relaxed.

- Support the scrotum and testicles in the palm of your hand, to feel their weight. One testicle may be slightly larger than the other, but they should be about the same weight.

- Hold a testicle between the thumb and fingers, with your thumb on top and first and second fingers underneath. Roll the testicle gently, feeling for any hard lumps. A normal testicle is oval in shape; it feels firm but not hard and is smooth with no lumps. Cancerous lumps are usually hard, on the front or side of a testicle, or may be a swelling of the testicle itself.

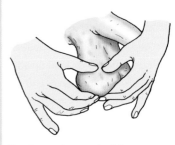

- Feel the epididymis, a sausage-shaped lump at the top and back of each testicle. It will feel soft and perhaps slightly tender.

How to examine your testicles

- Feel the spermatic cords which lead upwards from the epididymis and behind the testicles. They are firm, smooth tubes.

- Do the same with the other testicle. It would be very unusual to develop cancer in both testicles at the same time, so if you are not sure whether what you are feeling is normal, check it against the other side.

thread veins

Thread veins are tiny veins that appear most commonly on the cheeks, nose and legs. They have many names, including:

- spider veins
- broken veins
- capillary veins.

Normally, the tiny veins in the skin are invisible, but in some people they expand and show through the skin. One cause of this is too much exposure to the sun over the years. Another is pregnancy or estrogen treatment. They may also be inherited. Thread veins are more obvious after mid-life, when the skin becomes thinner and loses some of its collagen.

Treatments

Micro-sclerotherapy involves injecting the veins using tiny needles (like sclerotherapy for varicose veins described on page 189, but in miniature). This makes the walls of the veins stick together. If the therapist misses the tiny vein, and injects the surrounding skin by mistake, there can be a skin reaction. The thread veins may come back, but the treatment can be repeated.

Laser treatment gets rid of the veins very successfully, but can leave purplish bruises and tiny white scars. Some people find it painful, or notice a flicking sensation during the treatment. It is more expensive than sclerotherapy.

High-intensity light treatment (Photoderm) is a new method in which the veins are heated to make them coagulate. It can cover a bigger area than laser – areas measuring 2 cm by 0.5 cm can be treated by a single flash. There have been two scientific studies of the treatment, and they have given contradictory results. One study concluded that at least 75% of the veins were cleared in 80% of patients, and that after treatment the skin may look a little red and there may be some tiny blisters, but usually no scarring.

In the other study, patients found the treatment uncomfortable and described each light pulse as being like a burn. There was scarring and thinning of the skin in 21% of patients, and 42% had blistering and peeling. Only 9.5% of patients had complete clearance of the thread veins and there was no change in appearance in 56%. So, this technique appears to be more risky and less effective than laser treatment.

Electrolysis is cheap, and offered by many beauty clinics. It is less effective than the other treatments, and there is a greater risk of scarring.

Getting treatment

It may be difficult to get treatment for the thread veins through your doctor, because it comes into the 'cosmetic treatment' category. However, if you are very self-conscious about them, and find cover-up creams inadequate, it is worth asking your doctor. About a third of people with thread veins on the legs have varicose veins (see page 186); in this situation the varicose veins must be treated first.

You may have to use a private clinic. Clinics advertise persuasively, and it is difficult to know which provide good treatment. The best policy is to ask your doctor to find out the name of a good clinic from the local vascular surgeon. Before committing yourself to treatment, find out exactly what method the clinic uses, how many sessions will be needed and what the cost will be. Ask about problems, such as scarring. If laser is to be used, make sure it is not an older type – tunable dye or Yag – because these cause more scarring.

Self-help

You may find that alcoholic drinks, very hot drinks and spicy foods make the veins more obvious; if so, try to avoid them. Use a concealer cream under make-up. Horse chestnut cream (available from health food stores) is said to strengthen the tiny veins in the skin. Apply any skin cream gently to avoid traumatizing the skin.

Hormone replacement therapy (HRT) improves thread veins in some people (because it strengthens the skin slightly) but worsens them in others (because the estrogen in HRT encourages veins to dilate).

twitching eyes

"My eyes keep twitching – it looks as if I'm winking at people"

Uncontrollable twitching of the muscles round the eyes is called *blepharospasm* or *myokymia*. Only the eyelid may be affected, or the sufferer may keep blinking and closing the eyes repeatedly, or there may be spasms of not being able to open the eyes for a few moments or for longer periods. Sometimes the muscles of the lower face and the jaw are involved as well, so that trying to open the eyes causes these muscles to contract into a grimace. The twitching may be worse when the individual is tired or under stress, and it is often aggravated by bright or flickering light (such as that from a TV) or irritants such as smoke or wind.

Blepharospasm is not a dangerous condition, because it does not spread to other muscles of the body, but it can be embarrassing not to have control over one's facial expression. It is probably caused by a fault in the part of the brain that controls movements (the *basal ganglia*).

Although stress makes it worse, relaxation techniques do not seem to help. In fact, there is no cure, but it can be improved by tiny injections of botulinum toxin into the affected muscles. For this treatment, your doctor would have to refer you to a neurology department specializing in movement disorders. The treatment has to be repeated several times a year.

urinary incontinence

In women

"I sometimes wet myself when I cough or jump. And sometimes I suddenly need to go, and may not be able to get to the toilet in time"

- On average, about 2–3 pints of urine are produced by the kidneys every day
- Most people do not feel an urge to pass urine until there is about 150–200 ml in the bladder
- The normal adult bladder can hold about 500 ml (1 pint) of urine
- Four out of every 10 women have suffered from incontinence at some time in their adult life

Incontinence is leakage of urine from the bladder. It may be just a few drops or a dribble, or may be a stream. Incontinence is much more common than most people realize. A few years ago the UK broadcaster Claire Rayner spoke on TV about incontinence; afterwards, the program received more than 12,000 letters asking for more information. In fact, there are probably about 3 million people in Britain with this problem. It can happen to anyone at any age, but is more common in women. The idea that it affects only the elderly is completely out of date – the popularity of active sports, such as jogging, has caused more younger women to notice the problem. Incontinence is not a personal failure, nor is it something that 'women should expect'; in 70% of cases it can be cured.

How the bladder works
Each day, the kidneys empty about 3 pints of urine into the bladder. The wall of the

Percentage of women who have urinary incontinence	
Aged 15–44	5–7%
Aged 45–64	8–15%
Women aged over 65	About 15%

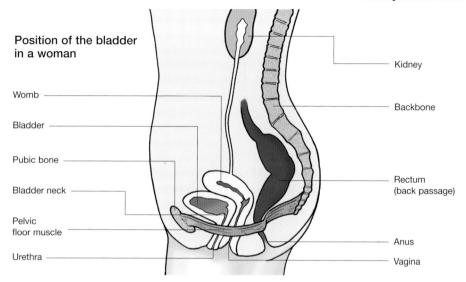

Position of the bladder in a woman

Womb

Bladder

Pubic bone

Bladder neck

Pelvic floor muscle

Urethra

Kidney

Backbone

Rectum (back passage)

Anus

Vagina

bladder is made of stretchy muscle, so that the bladder stretches like a balloon as it fills with urine.

A ring of muscle at the 'neck' of the bladder acts like a tap, keeping the urine in. This muscle is greatly strengthened by the muscles of the pelvic floor which stretch backwards from the pubic bone to the backbone. (The bowel, the vagina and the neck of the bladder pass through these *pelvic floor muscles*, which are normally kept firm and rather tense to hold the bowel, uterus and bladder in place.) In fact, without the help of the pelvic floor muscles, the bladder neck would not be able to keep the bladder closed.

When the bladder contains about a pint of urine, it signals to the brain that we need to urinate. When it is convenient for us to do so, the bladder muscle stops stretching and begins to contract, squeezing the urine out. At the same time, the bladder and pelvic floor muscles relax, allowing the urine out. The urine then passes down a short tube, called the urethra, to the outside.

Types of incontinence

Leaking of urine when you cough or laugh or bend over, or with exercise such as jumping or jogging, is called *stress incontinence*. It occurs if the muscles at the neck of the bladder are not strong enough to hold the urine in when the pressure in the abdomen is increased (as happens when you laugh or cough). No one knows why these muscles may become weak; some women notice the problem after childbirth or menopause. There is also some evidence that smoking weakens the pelvic floor. Suddenly needing to pass urine desperately, and maybe not being able to reach the toilet in time, is a slightly different sort of incontinence called *urge incontinence*. There are two main causes of urge incontinence. One is hypersensitivity of the bladder, so that it feels full when it isn't. The other is misbehavior of the bladder muscle: it starts to contract when it should be stretching to hold more urine. This is also called *irritable bladder*. It means that people with urge incontinence have to pass urine often (probably more than 8 times a day) but may not pass much each time.

Some people with incontinence have both stress incontinence and urge incontinence. The 'stress' symptoms may be more prominent than the 'urge' symptoms, or vice versa.

What you can do
Decide whether your problem is mainly stress incontinence or mainly urge incontinence.

For stress incontinence
- Some women find that wearing a sanitary tampon is helpful. The tampon should be a large size, or you can insert two smaller tampons side-by-side. In fact, the tampon in the vagina is supporting the bladder neck, which is in front and just above the vagina. You shouldn't wear a sanitary tampon all the time (because of the risk of toxic shock syndrome), but you can usually wear them for a short time (e.g. for an aerobics class).
- You can buy special devices to do the same job. The Conveen Continence Guard is an arch-shaped polyurethane foam device that you insert into the vagina; it has two wings to support the bladder neck. These devices can be left in for up to 16 hours, and do not need to be removed when you empty your bladder. They can be bought by mail order. These devices are disposable and expensive, but could be useful if you find stress incontinence a problem in certain situations, such as an aerobics class.
- The pelvic floor muscles can be strengthened by special exercises. These are very effective, and many people find they cure the problem completely. But they need patience to learn, and you may have to do them for a few months before you start to notice any improvement. One advantage is that they are invisible, so you can do them at any time – at bus stops, in the supermarket line, or while talking on the phone.
- Watch your weight – extra weight puts strain on the pelvic floor.

Pelvic floor exercises (especially useful for stress incontinence)

Learning the exercises

- Stand, sit or lie with your knees slightly apart. Now imagine that you are trying to stop yourself passing wind from the back passage: to do this you must tighten the muscles round the back passage. Squeeze and lift those muscles as if you really do have wind: you should be able to feel the muscles move and the skin round the back passage tightening. Your legs and buttocks should not move at all.

- Next, imagine that you are sitting on the toilet passing urine. Imagine yourself trying to stop the stream of urine (the stop test) – really try hard. You will be using the same group of muscles as in the first exercise, but you will find it more difficult.

- Next time you go to the toilet to pass urine, try the stop test about half way through emptying your bladder. (If the flow of urine speeds up you are using the wrong muscles.) Once you have stopped the flow of urine, relax and allow the bladder to empty completely. Don't worry if you find you can only slow up the stream, and cannot stop it completely.

- If you are unsure you are exercising the right muscles, put one or two fingers in the vagina and try the exercise to check. You should feel a gentle squeeze if you are exercising the pelvic floor. A common mistake is to just clench your buttocks and hold your breath; if you can't hold a conversation at the same time, you're doing the exercises wrongly. Don't tighten the tummy, thigh or buttock muscles or cross your legs. Only use your pelvic floor muscles.

Using pelvic floor exercises

- Do the stop test once a day while you are passing urine. **Do not** get into the habit of doing it every time you pass urine.

- Stand, sit or lie with your knees slightly apart. Slowly tighten and pull up the pelvic floor muscles as hard as you can: hold tightened for at least 5 seconds if you can, then relax (slow pull-up). Repeat at least five times. Now pull the muscles up quickly and tightly, then relax immediately (fast pull-up). Repeat at least five times. Do these exercises – five slow and five fast – at least ten times every day.

For urge incontinence

- The bladder can be 'retrained' to hold larger amounts of urine, so that the muscle doesn't start to contract until you are ready. This 'bladder retraining drill' is tedious but does work (see page 170).
- Don't get into the habit of going to the toilet 'just in case'; this encourages bladder misbehavior. Go only when you feel the bladder is full.

Bladder retraining drill
(especially useful for urge incontinence)

- Bladder retraining is based on passing urine by the clock at regular intervals.

- **Days 1 and 2:** start by choosing an interval you feel fairly confident you can achieve, such as $1^1/_2$ hours. Continue this for 2 days.

- **Days 3 and 4:** increase the interval between emptying by 15 minutes. Continue with this interval for 2 days.

- **Day 5 onwards:** when you are comfortable with the extra 15 minutes, increase it again. As each interval becomes manageable, increase it again.

- If holding on is difficult, distract yourself by watching TV or phoning a friend. You may find mental tricks helpful: for example, concentrate on the mental image of a tight knot in the neck of a balloon.

- It is natural to think that by cutting the amount you drink you will have more control. This is not true, and can even worsen the problem by increasing your susceptibility to irritating bladder infections (cystitis). However, it may be helpful to reduce the amount of tea, coffee or beer that you drink, replacing them with other drinks; the caffeine in tea and coffee can make the bladder irritable.

- Eat plenty of fresh fruit, vegetables and fiber to avoid constipation, which can press on the bladder and the urethra.

- Empty the bladder properly each time you pass urine; bending forward at the waist may help.

What your doctor can do
If you find that the exercises deal with the problem, there is probably no need to see the doctor. Otherwise, discuss it with your doctor, who will be able to check that you do not have an unusual type of incontinence. For example, you might have a prolapsed womb that is pressing on the bladder (see page 97).

Before you see the doctor, make a record for a day or two of how your bladder is actually behaving. Get a jug – one that you can easily pass urine into – marked in ml or fluid ounces, and use it to measure how much urine you pass on each occasion. Note down the time and the volume. Also note down any occasions when leakage occurs.

The doctor may wish to do a vaginal examination, inserting a speculum (like when you have a PAP smear) to check for prolapse of the womb.

The options

The doctor may then suggest any of the following options.

- Continue with the exercises, perhaps with the help of a specialist nurse. For example, the nurse may be able to provide special cones for you to insert in the vagina for a short period each day to strengthen the pelvic floor.

- It is possible to plug the urethra. Femassist is a small latex suction cap that is placed over the opening of the urethra (not inside). It helps to pull the walls of the urethra together, keeping it sealed until you remove it. It is easy to fit and remove making it cheaper than some other appliances. Appliances, such as Reliance and Autocath 100, are inserted into the urethra. These are slightly more tricky to use, and you will need to be shown how by a specialist nurse. They are suitable only for short periods, such as during exercise.

- Hormone replacement therapy (if you are near menopause). Some doctors think this may help both stress and urge incontinence, although there is little scientific evidence that it has any effect.

- For urge incontinence, some drugs can help but they all have side-effects. Propantheline (Pro-Banthine) is often used, but side-effects are dry mouth, blurred vision and constipation; oxybutynin (Ditropan or Cystrin) is more effective but the dry mouth or blurred vision are worse. Tolterodine (Detrusitol) is a new drug which is less likely to produce a dry mouth. Imipramine (Tofranil) and amitriptyline help urge incontinence by a different action from their antidepressant effect, and are particularly useful for women whose main problem is incontinence during orgasm (see page 175).

- If the cause of your incontinence is not obvious to the doctor, you may be referred to hospital for urodynamic tests to obtain an accurate diagnosis. These may cause some discomfort – a small tube (1 mm diameter) is inserted into the bladder to measure pressures, and sometimes a small tube is also inserted into the back passage.

- Collagen injections bulk up the tissues around the urethra and bladder neck, and are used for stress incontinence. The collagen is injected by inserting a needle alongside the urethra, or into the urethra and through its wall. A local anesthetic is given to prevent pain. Most women need two or three injections, at weekly intervals. About 60–70% of women find that their symptoms are cured or improved by the treatment, which is as effective in older women as it is in younger ones. However, the effect may not last, and 3 years later only 50% of people remain cured. For this reason (and because it's expensive), collagen injections are not often used in Europe, although they are popular in the US. Collagen injections have to be given by an expert, and you will need to have urodynamic tests first (see preceding page), which measure how your bladder is working.

- The collagen used in the injections comes from cattle hide taken from freshly slaughtered cattle. These cattle are bred and live in closed herds in the US, and never receive any animal protein in their diet. It is, therefore, very unlikely that collagen injections could transmit BSE. Some people are allergic to beef collagen, and everyone is given an allergy test 4 weeks before the injections are scheduled.
- Referral for a surgical operation. This is a last resort, and you would need urodynamic tests first. There are many different operations for stress incontinence (more than 100 at the last count). One of the best operations is *Burch retropubic colposuspension*. The success rate is about 90% but a few people are worse afterwards. Surgery cannot really help urge incontinence.

Living with incontinence

In a few cases, incontinence does not respond to treatment. In this situation, a wide range of disposable pads is available to suit individual needs. For example, a bulky pad may be best at night, and a less obtrusive pad might be preferable during the day. A very few people will require a catheter. This is a small tube passed into the bladder through the urethra. The urine empties down the catheter into a disposable bag that is secured to the thigh or waist and hidden under skirts or trousers.

In men

"I sometimes have to rush to the toilet to pass urine and I don't pass much when I get there: I thought it was only women who had that problem"

Incontinence or inability to control the passage of urine in men is usually caused by a blockage at the outlet of the bladder, caused by growth of the prostate gland. This condition is called *benign prostatic hyperplasia* (BPH). This tends to occur with aging.

Percentage of men who have urine incontinence	
Aged 15–64	5–7%
Aged 64 or over	10–20%

By the age of 60 years, about 40% of men have enlarged prostates, but this rises to 75% by the age of 80. The reason is not known, but it is not a cancerous condition.

A normal adult prostate is about the size of a golf ball and weighs 20–25 g (or about 1 ounce). With BPH it can increase to 60 g or more. As it expands, the prostate wraps itself round the neck of the bladder like a collar, restricting the outlet, and the bladder muscle has to work harder to push the urine out.

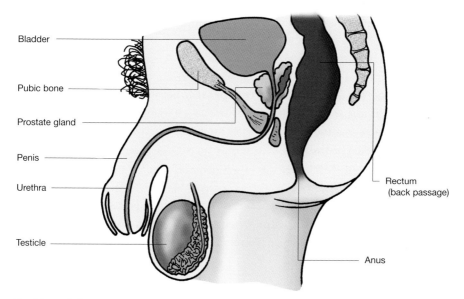

Bladder

Pubic bone

Prostate gland

Penis

Urethra

Testicle

Rectum (back passage)

Anus

Position of the prostate

You notice that you have a poor urine stream or that starting the stream is difficult or that urine seems to flow in stops and starts. Often the bladder feels incompletely empty after urination.

The strain makes the bladder muscle misbehave (see page 168), so that it often starts to contract before the bladder is full. This can happen quite suddenly, so you have to rush to the toilet to pass urine. If the contraction is large enough you may leak on the way – *urge incontinence*. This problem is often worse in cold weather or if you hear the sound of running water. Because the bladder tends to contract before it is full, you will pass urine frequently in small amounts and often have to get up in the night to urinate.

Questions to ask yourself if you think your prostate is enlarged

- Do you have difficulty in starting to pass urine?
- Do you think it takes you too long to pass urine?
- Do you pass urine in stops and starts?
- Do you dribble urine without full control when you have tried to stop?
- Do you have a sensation of not having emptied your bladder completely?
- Do you have to get up more than twice a night to pass urine, but only pass small amounts?
- Are you bothered by your waterworks?

If you answer 'yes' to any of these questions it is quite likely you have an enlarged prostate.

The bladder has difficulty in emptying completely, because the outlet is restricted, and there is always some urine left inside. Gradually the amount of urine remaining in the bladder increases and, in severe cases, eventually overflows without any feeling of urgency – *overflow incontinence.*

What you can do

There isn't much you can do to help yourself; bladder training drill (see page 170) is not very effective for men in this situation. You need to see your doctor. There is no need to be embarrassed; it is a common problem and around 350 000 men consult their doctors each year for this reason.

What your doctor can do

Your doctor needs to check that prostate enlargement is the cause of your symptoms. If the problem is really troubling you he or she may decide to try drug treatment. A drug (finasteride) is available to shrink the prostate. It may take 6 months or more to have its full effects, and if you stop taking it the prostate starts to grow again. Other drugs (alpha-blockers) relax the bladder neck and the prostate itself, and take only 4–6 weeks to have their full effects, but they have side-effects in some people. If the symptoms are bothersome and the obstruction severe, you may opt for a prostatectomy operation to remove the enlarged prostate.

urinating during sex

"I often pass urine while we're having sex: I can't control it"

- A doctor did a survey of women attending his urogynecology clinic (who of course already had an incontinence problem) and found that 24% had incontinence during intercourse. Most had felt too embarrassed to mention it to their doctor. Many women have leakage of urine during intercourse but not at any other time
- In about two-thirds, the leakage occurs when the penis enters the vagina (penetration)
- In about one-third, the leakage occurs only at orgasm

In 1950, a Dr Grafenberg described what he called *"female ejaculation*... the expulsion of large quantities of clear transparent fluid at the height of orgasm". Some sex manuals still talk about this female ejaculation as if it were some kind of discharge of sexual glands and link it to stimulation of the so-called G-spot in the vagina. This is complete rubbish; there is no evidence that this fluid is anything but urine.

Passing urine during intercourse, and being unable to control it, happens to many women. No one seems to talk about this, so a sufferer thinks she is the only one with the problem.

The reason is not understood, but it is likely to be partly due to an irritable bladder (see page 168) or a weakness at the neck of the bladder.

Treatment

Empty your bladder before sex. Your doctor may prescribe oxybutynin hydrochloride (2.5 mg or 5 mg) for you. You should take this about an hour before sex (if you can plan that well ahead!). Alternatively, your doctor can prescribe imipramine, to be taken in the evening. This is normally given as an antidepressant, but it also has effects on the bladder (which is why a similar drug is used to treat bed-wetting in children). If your doctor suggests it, it is because of its bladder effects, not because he or she thinks you are depressed. The dose will be lower than given for depression. Tolterodine (Detrusitol) is a newer drug with fewer side-effects.

If none of these deals with the problem, it would be worth seeing your gynecologist, preferably one who specializes in urogynecology. If you have leakage at other times, as well as during sex, an operation to strengthen the bladder neck is sometimes recommended. Unfortunately this operation is successful in controlling leakage during intercourse in only two-thirds of people.

In the end you and your partner may simply have to come to terms with the problem, and enjoy your sex life in spite of it. If it is causing a real problem in your relationship, or affecting your feelings about yourself, a few sessions with a psychosexual counselor can be very helpful (see page 135).

USEFUL CONTACTS

National Association For Continence, formerly Help for Incontinent People, is a not-for-profit organization dedicated to improving the quality of life of people with incontinence. NAFC's purpose is to be the leading source of education, advocacy and support to the public and to the health professional about the causes, prevention, diagnosis, treatments, and management alternatives for incontinence.

P.O. Box 8310
Spartanburg, SC 29305-8310
www.nafc.org
864-579-7900

vaginal problems

Vaginal discharge

It is normal to have some vaginal discharge. The vagina is naturally moist as part of its self-cleansing mechanism. This moist discharge clears dead cells and bacteria from the vagina. It comes mainly from glands in the cervix (neck of the womb). It is slightly acidic, which helps to keep infections at bay. The acidity is lactic acid, formed by 'friendly' bacteria as they break down sugars.

The amount of this normal discharge varies from woman to woman, and with the menstrual cycle. Many women notice that during the week after a period there is hardly any discharge, and what there is has a thick consistency. Towards the middle of the cycle (about 2 weeks after the start of a period) the amount increases and it becomes thin, slippery and clear, like uncooked egg white. When this discharge is exposed to the air it becomes brownish-yellow, so it is normal to find a yellowish stain on underwear at the middle of the monthly cycle. There may also be a feeling of moistness and stickiness. Discharge also increases during pregnancy. During sexual excitement, vaginal discharge becomes very profuse because two glands near the vaginal opening (Bartholin's glands) secrete additional slippery mucus, which acts as a lubricant for intercourse.

Normal discharge does not smell, and does not cause any irritation or itching.

A discharge is likely to be abnormal if:

- it smells fishy
- it is thick and white, like cottage cheese
- it is greenish and smells foul
- there is blood in it (except when you have your period)
- it is itchy
- you have any genital sores or ulcers
- you have abdominal pain or pain on intercourse
- it started soon after you had unprotected sex with someone you suspect could have a sexually transmitted disease.

If your discharge is thick and white and itchy it may be thrush, so you could try an anti-thrush cream or tablet from a pharmacist. If it has any other of the features listed above, you should go to your gynecologist.

Causes of abnormal discharge

Don't assume that a discharge is necessarily due to thrush; bacterial vaginosis is more common.

Bacterial vaginosis gives a fishy-smelling discharge, without any itching or soreness. It is discussed on page 194.

Thrush is caused by the yeast *Candida albicans*. About 1 in 5 women have *Candida* in the vagina, without it causing any symptoms. Hormones in the vaginal secretions and the 'friendly' vaginal bacteria keep it at bay. Problems arise when this natural balance is upset, and *Candida* multiplies. This can happen:

● during pregnancy
● when you take antibiotics (because these get rid of the friendly bacteria)

Myths about thrush

● **'The contraceptive pill causes thrush'**
Probably false. Doctors are still arguing about this, but there is very little evidence for it.

● **'Thrush is always a sexually transmitted disease'**
False. Women who are not sexually active can suffer from thrush. The *Candida* yeasts are already in the vagina, and they cause thrush when the body's natural balance that keeps it under control is upset.

● **'Thrush always causes a discharge'**
False. Itching is the usual symptom of thrush – there is often no discharge at all, or just a slight discharge.

● **'Thrush is very smelly'**
False. If there is an odor, it is minimal and not unpleasant.

● **'Thrush can be prevented by douching the vagina'**
Very definitely false. Douching is squirting a soapy or antiseptic solution into the vagina to 'cleanse' it. There is no need to do this, because the vagina cleans itself very efficiently. In fact, douching has the opposite effect; it destroys the 'friendly' bacteria, gets rid of the healthy acidity and damages the lining, allowing thrush and other infections to take hold easily.

- if you have diabetes, especially if your blood sugar levels are consistently too high
- if you wear tight, non-porous underwear, such as nylon underwear and tights (because *Candida* thrives in warm, moist conditions)
- if the vulva or vagina is sore for any other reason, particularly if you scratch (because damaged tissue is more susceptible to *Candida*)
- if you are ill for any reason
- if you are taking any drugs, such as steroids, which lower the body's resistance to infection.

Forgotten tampons are quite a common cause of discharge. It is easy to forget to remove the last tampon at the end of a period. After a week or two the tampon begins to fester, and there will be a foul-smelling discharge.

Gonorrhea is one of the most infectious sexually transmitted diseases. If a woman has unprotected sex with a man who has it, she has a 60–90% chance of catching it. It is caused by the *Gonococcus* bacteria. It is a serious infection, because if it is not treated it can spread upwards to the Fallopian tubes, and make the woman infertile. About 20% of women with gonorrhea have a foul-smelling, greenish-yellow discharge. About 20% have vague symptoms, such as a slight increase in discharge, pain on intercourse or lower abdominal discomfort. About 20% have no symptoms at all. (Most men with gonorrhea notice an obvious discharge – see page 113.)

Trichomonas is caused by a tiny amoeba-like (protozoan) organism called *Trichomonas vaginalis*. It used to be common, but for mysterious reasons is becoming less so; over

Type of discharge	Possible causes
Thick and white	Normal in some women Thrush (*Candida*)
Itchy	Thrush (*Candida*) *Trichomonas*
Smelly	Bacterial vaginosis *Trichomonas* Gonorrhea Forgotten tampon

the last 10 years the number of cases in England and Wales has fallen from 17,000/year to 5,000/year. It causes a discharge that is often frothy and yellowish-greenish, but it may be thin and scanty. The discharge is smelly, and the vulva is often sore. It may also be painful to pass urine. It is caught from a man who has it, but he may be unaware of his condition as most men with *Trichomonas* don't have any symptoms. It is not dangerous, although some doctors think it could possibly spread to the Fallopian tubes.

Tests that may be needed

The doctor will look at the vulva for any signs of thrush, and will then insert a metal device called a speculum into the vagina so that the inside of the vagina can be inspected. Samples of the discharge can be taken by wiping with cotton-wool swabs. A doctor will usually have to send the swabs to a laboratory, so it may be some days before the result is available. A clinic can look at the samples under the microscope straight away, and can usually tell you the diagnosis within half an hour, though they are also sent to the main laboratory for confirmation. Don't be surprised if you see the doctor or nurse testing the acidity of the discharge with litmus paper, or mixing some of it with a liquid (potassium hydroxide) on a glass slide and then sniffing it; these are standard tests for bacterial vaginosis.

Treatments and self-help:

- Even if you are fairly sure it is thrush, don't persist with an anti-thrush cream from the pharmacist if it doesn't resolve the problem in a day or two, or if the discharge returns; go to a clinic and get a proper diagnosis.
- Each cause has its own proper treatment, and it is important to follow the treatment instructions from the clinic very carefully. If the clinic asks you to return for another check-up it is important that you do so, even if the discharge has gone. The clinic may be checking for gonorrhea, which can damage your Fallopian tubes and infect a future sexual partner without you having any further symptoms.
- If you have thrush, try to avoid the situations listed on pages 178–179 which encourage it. Also:
  - dry the vulval area carefully after washing
  - avoid bubble baths and scented soaps and don't put any disinfectants in the bath
  - shower well after swimming in a chlorinated pool and don't sit around in a wet bathing suit

- wear cotton underwear
- change your underwear after exercising
- don't use 'enzyme' or 'biological' washing powders for your underwear
- change tampons or sanitary pads frequently (2–3 times a day).

● Ask your partner to go to a clinic for a check-up if your doctor advises he does so, or if he has any discharge from the urethra (the opening at the end of the penis) or any soreness or irritation of the penis.

Dry vagina

"My dry vagina is really uncomfortable, especially during sex"

● Natural vaginal moisture cleans the vagina; it clears away all the blood within 24 hours of finishing a period

● Before menopause, 16% of women have vaginal dryness

● Vaginal dryness is more of a problem after menopause, when about 45% of women suffer from it

● Vaginal dryness seems to be more common in women who have had a hysterectomy (even if they still have their ovaries)

The vagina is normally moist inside. This prevents the sides of the vagina rubbing against each other as you move about during the day. The vaginal moisture is slightly acidic, which helps to keep infections such as thrush at bay. This acidity is due to the 'friendly' bacteria that live in the vagina and help to keep it healthy.

Vaginal moisture is mainly produced by the cervix (neck of the womb) at the top of the vagina and eventually oozes out of the vagina – some vaginal discharge is normal (see page 177). This means that there is a very slow flow of moisture through the vagina, and this keeps it clean, taking dead cells and the remains of the menstrual period to the outside.

When you are sexually excited, two special glands at the entrance of the vagina, called *Bartholin's glands*, produce extra secretions. The moisture from Bartholin's glands is more slimy than the moisture from the cervix, because its purpose is to provide good lubrication during intercourse. Its musky smell is the result of millions of years of evolution to increase female attractiveness to the male of the species, by signalling that she is ready for sex.

How the vagina lubricates and cleans itself

Womb

Cervix

Cervix produces moist secretions

Wall of vagina

Secretions flow downwards, cleaning and lubricating the vagina

Bartholin's gland

During sexual excitement, extra lubrication is provided by the Bartholin's glands

Normal discharge gets rid of dead cells, harmful bacteria and remains of menstrual blood

Dryness before menopause

Vaginal dryness before menopause is mostly a problem during sex. It may mean that you are not sufficiently aroused – which can occur for all sorts of reasons such as inadequate foreplay, guilt, fear or relationship problems. Male arousal is often ahead of female arousal, so your partner may be attempting penetration before good lubrication has occurred. Lack of lubrication is common in breast-feeding women, because estrogen levels are low.

A dry vagina can be lubricated easily. For additional lubrication for intercourse, use a water-soluble, starch-based lubricant – such as KY Jelly, Replens or Senselle – rather than a petroleum-based product like Vaseline which may interfere with your natural secretions. Some lubricants damage rubber/latex condoms; KY, Replens and Senselle do not.

- KY is used just before intercourse. Smear it liberally over the vulval area, especially round the opening of the vagina.
- Replens and Senselle are artificial lubricants which you use two or three times a week. They coat the inside of the vagina with a non-hormonal moisturizer which lasts for a day or two, so they do not have to be used immediately before intercourse.

These lubricants can be bought from a pharmacist; you do not need a prescription.

Dryness after menopause

Vaginal dryness can be a particular problem at and after menopause, due to lack of estrogen (the female hormone). Estrogen is responsible for the plumpness of the lining of the vagina, for the elasticity of the tissues round the vagina and for the production of the moisture from the cervix. Estrogen levels fall at menopause, so the vagina loses some of its elasticity, its lining becomes thinner, and it feels dryer. Because there is less moisture, there are fewer of the 'friendly' bacteria that help to keep the vagina acidic. When the vagina becomes less acid, infections such as thrush can take hold, which cause further irritation and discomfort.

All these changes can make intercourse uncomfortable. Another factor is that after the menopause Bartholin's glands are less efficient – they take longer to produce the lubricating juices for sex, and produce less than in younger women. The American sex researchers Masters and Johnson showed that whereas younger women may become sufficiently aroused for penetrative sex in as short a time as a few seconds, the menopausal women may take 5 minutes or more.

Treatments

HRT (hormone replacement therapy) will increase vaginal lubrication and thicken the vaginal lining, as well as dealing with hot flushes and preventing osteoporosis (thinning of the bones).

A vaginal estrogen cream can be prescribed by your doctor if you prefer not to take HRT. For the first 2 or 3 weeks you use this every night, and it may be a week or two before you notice any improvement. After that, twice a week will be enough.

The creams can be messy. Some come with a special syringe (applicator) to help you insert the cream into the vagina. In fact, applicators are more trouble than they are worth, because they have to be washed in warm soapy water after each use. More importantly, they tend to give you too much cream. Some of the estrogen will then be absorbed through the vaginal wall into the bloodstream, where it could be harmful.

Unless you have had a hysterectomy, estrogen in the bloodstream needs to be balanced by progesterone tablets, otherwise there is a slight risk of cancer of the womb. Hormone replacement tablets provide both estrogen and progesterone, but vaginal cream contains only estrogen. If you use too much of the cream you are putting estrogen without progesterone into the bloodstream. To be on the safe side, some doctors prescribe progesterone tablets for women using estrogen vaginal cream.

It is better to smear the cream inside the vagina with your fingers, and not to be over-lavish. If you are not used to touching the inside of your vagina you may find this peculiar at first, but you will very soon become relaxed about doing so.

Vaginal estrogen tablets (Vagifem) are another possibility. They need a doctor's prescription. Each tablet comes in an applicator which is about the size of a pencil. You insert the applicator into the vagina and press the end to release the tablet into the vagina. For the first 2 weeks you use one tablet a day, but later only two a week are needed.

An estrogen-containing vaginal ring (Estring) may be suggested by your doctor. This gradually releases estrogen into the vagina. It has to be replaced every 3 months, and you must not use it for more than 2 years in total. It is not painful or uncomfortable, although there is sometimes slight irritation at first. Some people find that it gets in the way during intercourse, in which case you can remove it beforehand and put it back afterwards. It is easy to take in and out – your doctor will show you how.

Leisurely sex with lots of foreplay is particularly important for the older woman. This allows Bartholin's glands to produce the maximum amount of juice before penetration.

Simple lubricants such as KY, Replens or Senselle can be used if you need additional lubrication for intercourse.

vaginal lips

"The lips of my vagina hang down – I feel a freak"

The outer vaginal lips are usually fleshy, and the inner lips are usually thin but, like every other part of the body, they come in all shapes and sizes. In some women, the inner lips are completely enclosed by the outer lips. In other women, the inner lips hang down further than the outer ones, but this is absolutely normal. But, if the inner lips are so large that they are upsetting you, it is possible to have them trimmed by a surgical operation.

What to do

It would be best to start by visiting your gynecologist. Explain to the doctor that you have not come for tests, but because you have another worry. You can then ask the doctor to examine your vaginal lips, and tell you whether or not they are abnormally large. The advantage of going to the gynecologist is that these doctors examine dozens of women every day, so they will be able to give you a good opinion. If the doctor says that you are unusual, you can then ask to arrange for an operation if you wish.

varicose veins

- One person in five has varicose veins or is likely to get them
- Varicose veins usually develop slowly over 10–20 years
- Men as well as women can have varicose veins, but they are six times more common in women
- Varicose veins are the price we pay for our upright posture: if we still walked on all fours they probably wouldn't occur
- 50,000 Britons have hospital treatment for varicose veins every year

A bulging section of blue, twisted vein on the back of a person's calf or thigh is a common sight. A varicose vein is actually a vein that has lost its elasticity. Its wall has become flabby, so that it easily becomes swollen with blood.

How normal veins function

As the heart beats, it propels blood containing oxygen into the arteries. The arteries deliver this blood around the body to the muscles and organs. When it reaches the muscles and organs, oxygen is removed from the blood. This 'used' blood is then returned to the heart in the veins so that the cycle can begin again. It is the pumping action of the heart that keeps blood moving through the arteries. However, by the time the blood reaches the veins, the force behind the blood is reduced, as the blood has already travelled a long way. The veins in the leg have a particular problem in getting the blood back to the heart, because they have to carry the blood uphill, against the force of gravity. But the body has a mechanism to deal with the situation. It consists of the following two elements.

- Some of the leg veins are deep in the muscle. These are called the *deep veins*. The contractions of the leg muscles during walking squeeze these veins, forcing blood along; this is called the *muscle pump*.
- To prevent the blood going backwards, and away from the heart, veins have one-way *valves*.

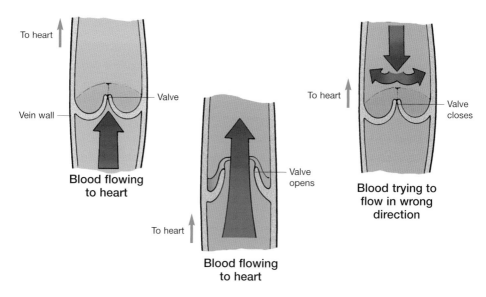

Not all the veins in the leg lie in the muscle like the deep veins; some are nearer the surface of the leg, in the skin and fatty tissue outside the muscle. These are called *superficial veins*. There are junctions between the deep veins and those outside the muscle. Each junction has a valve, which ensures that blood flows from the vein outside the muscle into the deep vein, and not back the other way. Once it is in a deep vein, blood can be pushed up to the heart by the muscle pump.

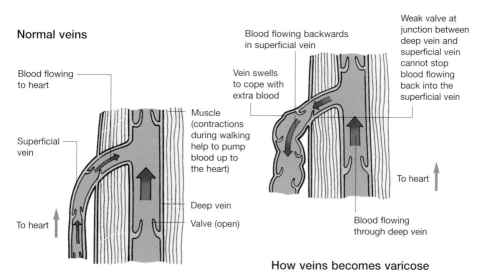

How veins becomes varicose

How varicose veins form

It is the veins that lie outside the muscle, not the deep veins that become varicose. The basic cause is failure of the valves at the junctions between these two types of veins. If one of these valves becomes weak it will allow blood to flow back into the vein outside the muscle. Over a period of time, this vein will swell to cope with the extra blood, lose its elasticity and become a lumpy, blue, varicose vein. The swelling means that the next valve below will eventually be unable to close, because its edges will no longer meet each other in the closed position. So there is a domino effect, with each damaged vein eventually producing damage to the one below it. As it does so, more of the vein will swell and become varicose. This happens very slowly over years.

Who gets varicose veins

Varicose veins affect both men and women, and are more likely with increasing age. They tend to run in families. They may first occur during pregnancy because of hormonal changes that relax the wall of the vein and because of pressure in the veins from the expanding uterus (womb). After the baby is born, there will be a general improvement in the veins, but they often become worse again in later pregnancies. Obesity and repeated abdominal strain (for example, from heavy lifting) may contribute. Long periods of standing and sitting with the legs bent and crossed makes them worse. Sometimes they occur after a serious *thrombosis* (blood clot) in the deep veins, because this may damage the valves at the main junctions.

It has been suggested that a diet low in fiber increases the likelihood of varicose veins (because if we are constipated we have to strain to open our bowels, which puts pressure on the veins), but this is unproven.

Symptoms of varicose veins

Varicose veins are a problem for three reasons.

- They look ugly. Because the affected veins are just below the skin, the enlarged and twisted portions are very obvious.
- The pools of non-circulating blood cause symptoms. Varicose veins often ache, sometimes itch or tingle, and usually cause swelling and pain in the feet and ankles. Some people have cramps and a feeling of restlessness in the legs.
- Bad varicose veins over many years can damage the skin near the ankle – the skin becomes stained brownish-black, and ulcers may occur which are difficult to heal.

How you can help yourself

- Take regular walks. Walking is the best exercise to improve the flow of blood in the legs.
- Avoid long periods of standing. If you have to stand in one position for longer than a few minutes, do some ankle movements, such as standing on tiptoe to encourage your calf muscles to pump blood out of your leg veins.
- Put your feet up whenever you are sitting around at home. This will help the veins to empty, and reduce swelling of the feet. Try not to cross your legs, or to sit for long periods with your legs bent. On long train or plane journeys, walk around from time to time; and on long car or train journeys take advantage of any stops to get out and walk for a few minutes.
- Don't wear garters or tight 'hold-up' stockings.
- Eat a healthy diet with lots of fruit and vegetables, to avoid constipation.
- Take extra care of the skin on your legs. If you have varicose veins, the blood stagnates and the circulation to the skin is poor. The skin can become deprived of oxygen and any damage will take longer to heal. Use a moisturizing lotion, don't scratch any itchy areas, try to avoid knocks and don't toast your legs in front of a fire.

When to ask for treatment

Don't feel you are wasting your doctor's time if you request treatment for veins that are not too bad. Surgeons prefer to deal with early cases because they are easier, and because the results are better. Color changes in the skin caused by varicose veins never completely reverse after surgery.

It used to be said that women who develop varicose veins after pregnancy should not be treated if they intend to have more children. Most surgeons now believe it is best to treat after the first baby, rather than wait until the woman's family is complete.

Treatments for varicose veins

Elastic stockings are often used when the varicose veins are likely to be temporary (for example during pregnancy). It is important that they are put on immediately after rising in the morning before blood and fluid have pooled in the feet and ankles.

Sclerotherapy consists of injecting a solution into the varicose vein. The solution causes irritation, inflammation, and eventually scarring, which permanently blocks the vein. The body absorbs the accumulated blood from the varicose vein, and the lumps flatten out over time.

Surgery often involves tying off the vein *(ligation)* above the varicose section, usually just before it joins the deep vein. The vein can be removed by *stripping* – one end of a tiny wire is attached at the varicose section, the other end is threaded through the vein to a small incision at the calf or ankle where the wire, along with the varicose section of vein, is pulled out.

Varicose vein surgery used to cause horrendous bruising, but now that doctors use fine instruments which need only tiny incision there should be little bruising. However, some surgeons still make big cuts in the legs, so ask about this before you decide to have the operation. You can usually leave the hospital on the day of operation or the following morning and then go back to work 1–2 days later (unless your work involves standing, in which case you would need a week off). The leg is bandaged for the first 12 hours, and then a heavy elastic stocking is worn. You may need painkillers for a few days after the operation.

A newer type of surgery is called SEPS, which is short for *subfascial endoscopic perforating vein surgery*. In this operation, the communicating veins with the ineffective valves that are causing the problem, are closed off.

Sclerotherapy versus surgery. The surgeon will decide whether sclerotherapy or surgery is better in an individual case. It depends on where the leaky valves are, and whether there are any problems in other veins. This can be assessed by *Doppler ultrasound,* a painless test which listens to sound waves reflected from the moving blood.

Some surgeons use a hand-held Doppler machine. Gently squeezing the calf will produce a 'whoosh' as the blood flows upwards in the veins above. Normally this is followed by silence as the valves close to prevent the blood flowing back down; if the surgeon hears the noise of blood flow, the valves are not working properly in that position. This method can be used to test the veins at various places in the leg.

A more sophisticated version of the technology is known as *color duplex sonography.* It displays a picture of the blood flow on a screen – forward flow as red and backward flow as blue – and is used for difficult cases, because it shows the deeper veins of the leg.

In general

- If there is damage to the valves at the junctions of the deep veins, surgery will be needed; this is usually the case if there are varicose veins in the thigh.
- Less severe varicose veins can be treated by sclerotherapy.

The body does not miss veins that are blocked with sclerotherapy or removed by surgery. The legs have many alternative veins for the blood to flow through. Problems never return in properly treated veins, but other veins can still become varicose.

USEFUL CONTACTS
Varicose Veins : A Guide to Prevention and Treatment
by Howard C. Baron, Barbara A. Ross (Facts on File)

vulva

Itchy vulva

The vulva is the fleshy area that surrounds the vaginal opening. Itching of the vulva io almost never caused by a sexually transmitted disease. It is usually either thrush or a skin condition. The lips of the vulva are covered by ordinary skin, so it can be affected by skin disorders, such as eczema and psoriasis, like any other part of the body. Sometimes the vulva may be the only part of the body to be affected, so you may be surprised by the diagnosis. Some of these skin disorders can be very itchy.

The usual mistake with vulval itching is to assume it is thrush, and to keep applying anti-thrush creams from the pharmacist. After a while these creams may even worsen the problem, because it is possible to develop an allergy to some of the ingredients. If an anti-thrush cream doesn't deal with the problem within a few days, or if the itching comes back, see your doctor. If the cause is actually a skin condition, not thrush, you need the appropriate treatment.

Thrush doesn't always cause a discharge; the main symptom is itching or soreness, worse in the week before a period. If there is a discharge it is usually only slight and non-smelly, and looks like cottage cheese (see page 178).

Psoriasis is a skin condition which can be extremely itchy in the genital area. It is usually bright red, often with painful cracks. It may extend to the groin, and to around the back passage (anus) and between the buttocks. Psoriasis on other parts of the body is scaly (check your scalp, knees and elbows), but in the vulval area it tends to be smooth. You can have psoriasis on the vulva without having it anywhere else on the body.

Lichen sclerosis is another extremely itchy skin condition of the vulva. The itching is often so bad that it prevents sleep. It is most common around menopause and in girls just before puberty, although it can occur at any age. The cause is a mystery. The skin looks thin and pale, and the area round the anus is often affected as well. If it is not treated, after some years the lips of the vulva shrink and the opening of the vagina narrows, so that sexual intercourse becomes painful. Treatment is simple, and your doctor can prescribe a special steroid cream.

Allergies and sensitivities can cause redness and itching. The vulval area seems to be very sensitive to chemicals, probably because the vulva is moist and warm which helps chemicals to penetrate the skin. It is possible to develop an allergy to almost any chemical substance that comes into contact with the vulva: skin creams (including anti-thrush creams); perfumes in soaps, shower gels, bubble baths and shampoos; disinfectants; fabric softeners and detergents; deodorant sprays (including 'intimate' deodorants).

What you can do
Start by trying to eliminate anything that could be causing an allergy or sensitivity. Stop using bubble bath or shower gel; use only a non-perfumed soap. Don't put disinfectant in the bath. Don't shampoo your hair in the bath, or in the shower where the shampoo could run down and be trapped in the vulval skin folds. Don't use 'intimate' deodorants, or apply deodorant or perfume to sanitary towels. Use a detergent labelled 'for sensitive skin' for washing your underwear and don't use fabric softener. Don't go swimming while you have the irritation – the chlorine may make it worse.

Soothe the skin by adding two handfuls of ordinary kitchen salt to your bath, or by bathing the area with salt solution (a heaped tablespoon of kitchen salt in a sinkful of warm water).

If you think thrush is a possibility, buy an anti-thrush cream from the pharmacist. This should work within a day or two. If it doesn't, or if the itching soon returns, see your doctor. This is a common symptom which your doctor deals with all the time, so there is no need to feel awkward. (Also see page 9 about getting help for a genital problem.)

White vulva
The vulva is normally slightly darker than the rest of your skin – dusky-pink or brownish. There are two conditions in which it becomes white in color.

Lichen sclerosis is described on the opposite page. In lichen sclerosis the vulva is usually itchy as well as pale. It needs treatment, so see your doctor.

Vitiligo. In this condition the normal skin pigment is lost from patches of skin, so the patches become milky-white. If your skin is naturally dark, vitiligo will be very obvious. The texture of the skin is normal and it is not painful or itchy. It may affect other parts of your body as well, or the vulva may be the only site. Vitiligo often runs in families, and usually appears in the teens. It is probably an *autoimmune disorder,* caused by the body making antibodies against its own pigment cells. It is not known why it affects some parts of the body (such as the genitals, face, hands and feet) more than others.

Vitiligo on other parts of the body can be treated with ultraviolet light, usually two or three times a week for at least 6 months. This usually produces some repigmentation of the area. When it affects only the genital area it is not usually treated, but if you are very distressed by it ask your doctor for a referral to a dermatologist.

Fishy-smelling vulva

If your vulva smells fishy, it is almost certain that you have *bacterial vaginosis* (also known as *anaerobic vaginosis*). The smell is often worse after sex, and during your period. There will usually be a discharge from the vagina as well as the fishy smell. The discharge is watery and a greyish, off-white color. It does not cause soreness or irritation. Bacterial vaginosis is common; in 1994, more than 37,000 women attending clinics in the UK had this problem.

The cause is an imbalance in the bacteria in the vagina. All women normally have some harmless bacteria in the vagina. In bacterial vaginosis, some of these multiply so that greater than normal numbers are present – mainly *Gardnerella* and *Mobiluncus* bacteria. In other words, bacterial vaginosis is not an infection caught from a sexual partner; these bacteria are normally present in the vagina.

Bacterial vaginosis is easily treated with an antibiotic called metronidazole. This cures the problem in 90% of women. Metronidazole causes an unpleasant metallic taste in the mouth, but this disappears after the course of treatment is finished. It can also cause a slight feeling of nausea, and you must avoid alcohol while taking it. An alternative is clindamycin cream, inserted into the vagina, but this may result in thrush. Ofloxacin, another antibiotic, can be used, but is not as effective as metronidazole.

Unfortunately, the cure may not be permanent. The problem recurs in about 50% of people. Your doctor may repeat the metronidazole treatment, or may try another antibiotic. Alternatively, try acetic acid vaginal jelly (Aci-Jel), which can be bought from a pharmacy without prescription. The pack contains a special applicator for inserting the jelly into the vagina; one applicatorful is used twice a day. It restores the natural acidity of the vagina, which encourages the natural balance of bacteria in the vagina and discourages the overgrowth of *Gardnerella* and *Mobiluncus*. There is no evidence that treating your sexual partner makes any difference.

In the past, bacterial vaginosis was thought to be just a nuisance, and not harmful in any way. There is now evidence that it doubles the likelihood of preterm labor, so if you are intending to become pregnant you should have bacterial vaginosis treated beforehand. (Metronidazole should not be used during pregnancy.) It may also increase the risk of pelvic inflammatory disease, which is infection of the Fallopian tubes.

Other vulval problems: see pages 78, 126, 178, 185.

wind (farting & belching)

- At any one time, there is about 200 ml (a mugful) of gas in the gut
- Most people expel about 600 ml of gas/day, but some people produce up to 2 liters
- Gut gases are 90% nitrogen; the remainder is carbon dioxide, hydrogen, methane and sometimes hydrogen sulphide
- Healthy young men break wind 14–25 times a day

Everyone's gut contains gas because:

- we cannot help swallowing air when we swallow food, when we drink and when we swallow our saliva
- carbon dioxide is produced by chemical reactions within the gut. (Saliva contains bicarbonate, which reacts with acid in the stomach to produce carbon dioxide gas; stomach acid also releases carbon dioxide when it reacts with pancreatic digestive juices in the upper part of the intestine.)
- the gases hydrogen, methane and carbon dioxide are produced by bacteria acting on food residues in the large bowel.

Some of the intestinal gas is absorbed into the bloodstream and is eventually exhaled by the lungs. However, most has to be got rid of through the mouth (belching, eructation) or through the anus (flatulence, farting, breaking wind). Nitrogen, carbon dioxide and hydrogen are odorless; hydrogen sulphide and methane smell bad. Some experts believe that our attempts to hold gas in are an unnatural result of our enclosed lifestyles and the build-up of pressure is responsible for bowel diseases such as diverticulosis – when we lived mainly in the open air farting was not a problem, and no one was worried about letting wind pass out naturally. In the early 1990s a publicity campaign was launched in Holland (by the National Liver and Intestine Foundation) to encourage people to break wind at least 15 times a day.

Reasons for farting and belching

Flatulent foods. Onions, tomatoes and mints actually relax the muscle at the lower end of the gullet, allowing air from the stomach to escape by belching.

Foods with a high proportion of unabsorbable carbohydrates that cause flatulence

- Beans
- Peas
- Broccoli, cauliflower
- Artichokes and other root vegetables such as parsnips
- 'Slimming foods' containing sorbitol or fructose
- Raisins, prunes
- Apples

Farting is more to do with bacteria in the lower bowel, which are particularly partial to carbohydrates. The carbohydrates in some foods cannot be broken down and absorbed in the intestine; they pass straight through to the bowel, where they are fermented by the bacteria to produce gas which comes out as farting. Beans are famous for containing large amounts of 'unabsorbable carbohydrate' but other foods can have the same effect.

Some slimming chocolate contains sorbitol or fructose instead of sugar. Most of this is not absorbed (which is why these products are marketed for dieters), but can be acted on by the large bowel bacteria.

Overeating, as we all know, leads to belching. This is because the stomach normally contains some air. When we overeat, the stomach attempts to relieve the discomfort and distension by expelling the stomach air upwards. This is a reflex over which we have no control.

Carbonated drinks, and gulping of hot drinks, introduces gas into the stomach.

Habit leads some people to suck a small amount of air into the esophagus or stomach by swallowing to make themselves belch, without realizing they are doing so. This habit often starts if there is a period of indigestion, when belching may temporarily relieve the discomfort.

Smoking, chewing gum and sucking on pen tops makes you produce more saliva which has to be swallowed. Each time you swallow the saliva you also swallow air.

The digestive system

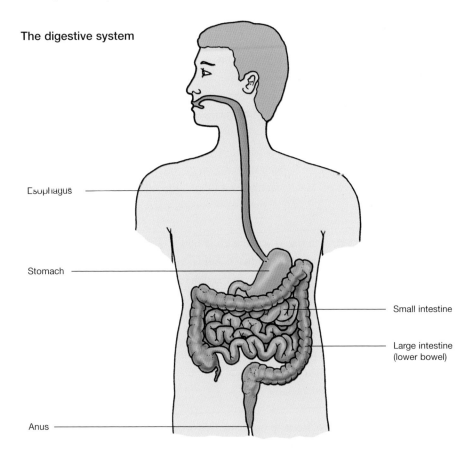

Esophagus

Stomach

Small intestine

Large intestine
(lower bowel)

Anus

Acarbose (Glucobay) is a drug for diabetes. It prevents enzymes in the gut digesting carbohydrates such as starch and sucrose. Because they are not digested, these carbohydrates are not absorbed (which is how the drug helps to lower the blood sugar). Instead, they pass down to the lower bowel, where they are fermented by the bacteria. Most people taking acarbose experience flatulence, tummy rumbles and a feeling of fullness.

Intestinal diseases are occasionally responsible. In lactose deficiency, for example, there is a deficiency of the enzyme that breaks down lactose, a carbohydrate found in milk. The undigested lactose produces hydrogen and carbon dioxide when it reaches the large bowel, causing frothy diarrhea, griping pains and flatulence.

Constipation can cause farting. Normally, most of the intestinal gas is expelled out of the anus as small puffs which we are not aware of. When we are constipated the gas becomes trapped behind the feces, and then suddenly emerges as a noticeable amount. Also, when we are constipated the food residues stay in the bowel for longer, and have more time to ferment and give off gases.

Anxiety and tension seem to make wind worse. This is partly because when we are anxious we are hyper-alert, and notice body functions that we would otherwise ignore. Another factor is that when we are anxious we tend to swallow more air. Also, our guts become more active because of increased adrenaline levels and they expel the gases more forcefully.

After childbirth: childbirth can damage the muscles of the anus or the nearby nerves, making it difficult to hold wind in. If your problem started after having a baby, see your doctor because an operation may cure the problem.

Aging may make gas worse because as we get older we do not produce digestive juices, such as saliva, as efficiently. This means that more carbohydrate foods pass untouched to the lower bowel, where they are fermented by the bacteria.

When wind is serious
Wind is never serious, except as a cause of embarrassment, unless there are other gut symptoms as well, such as abdominal pain, constipation, loss of weight, pale feces which are difficult to flush away, or blood in the feces.

Minimizing wind
- Try to avoid large quantities of the particular gas-forming foods listed on page 197, but make sure you eat enough fruit and vegetables to avoid constipation and give yourself a balanced diet. The carbohydrates in many foods (such as potatoes, rice, corn and wheat products) are well absorbed so will not worsen flatulence. Dietary fiber such as bran and cellulose are also innocent, because they are not converted to gases by gut bacteria.
- Don't suddenly increase the amount of fiber in your diet; the gut needs to get used to increased fiber gradually.
- Avoid carbonated drinks and hot drinks.

- Don't rush your food. When you gulp food you swallow more air.
- Don't overeat. To avoid gas it is better to eat little and often.
- Chew your food properly. This helps the saliva to work on it so it is properly digested, and you are less likely to swallow air with food that is chewed small than with large lumps.
- Avoid 'slimming' foods containing sorbitol.
- Remove 80% of the most troublesome carbohydrates from dried beans by covering them with water, bringing them to the boil and boiling for 10 minutes, turning off the heat and letting them soak for 4 hours. Drain off the water, replace with fresh water and cook the beans according to your recipe.
- Stop smoking.
- Do not use chewing gum, and try to avoid sucking on pen tops.
- Get plenty of exercise. This helps to keep the bowel moving normally.
- Try taking a charcoal tablet (such as JL Braggs' Medicinal Charcoal, available from pharmacies), or eating a charcoal biscuit (available from health food stores) before a meal.
- Your doctor might be willing to give you a course of broad-spectrum antibiotic. This can sometimes help by changing the balance of bacteria in the gut.

Disguising wind

If you make a smell in the lavatory, light a match – this makes the smell disappear as if by magic. Considerate people keep a box of matches by the lavatory for this purpose.

ZZZzzzzzz_{zzz}

See **Snoring** page 145

Glossary

A **Abscess:** a cavity or hollow space containing pus

Acne: a skin disorder, in which there are pustules and blackheads

Alopecia: the medical word for baldness (from the Greek word *alopekia*, meaning 'fox-mange')

Alopecia areata: a type of baldness in which hair is lost completely from a round patch

Alopecia totalis: loss of all the hair on the scalp

Alopecia universalis: loss of all the body hair as well as the scalp hair

Anal canal: the passage which feces pass along. It is made of rings of muscle, is about 4 cm (1½ inches) long, and connects the rectum to the anal opening

Anal sphincter: the rings of muscle in the anal canal that keep the feces in until we are ready to defecate

Androgens: hormones that are present in men and women, but more so in men (for example, testosterone)

Anaerobic vaginosis: bacterial vaginosis

Anus: the opening of the gut at its lower end, through which we pass stools

Areola: the pinkish-brown area surrounding the nipple in both men and women

B **Bacterial vaginosis:** an imbalance of bacteria in the vagina. There is usually a discharge from the vagina and the vulva is fishy-smelling

Balanitis: inflammation of the head (glans) of the penis

Balanitis xerotica obliterans: a skin condition of the penis. The foreskin becomes pale and thickened

Bartholin's glands: these glands are just inside the opening of the vagina, one on each side. They help produce lubrication for sex

Benign prostatic hyperplasia (BPH): non-cancerous enlargement of the prostate gland

Bladder neck: the exit of the bladder into the urethra, which is the tube through which we pass urine

Blepharospasm: uncontrollable twitching of the muscles around the eyes

Burch retropubic colposuspension: an operation for stress incontinence

C ***Candida:*** a type of fungus that can cause infections

Circumcision: a surgical operation on the penis to remove the foreskin

Cyclical breast pain: breast pain related to the menstrual cycle – it is common to have painful breasts before a period

D **Deep veins:** veins that lie in the muscles

Dermabrasion: procedure in which the skin is 'planed down' using a high-speed wire brush

Dermatologist: doctor specializing in illnesses of the skin, hair and nails

Detrusor muscle: the muscle of the wall of the bladder

Dyspareunia: painful sex

E **Ejaculation:** the peak of male orgasm, when the semen spurts out

Emergency contraception: prevents pregnancy after sex

Endoscopic transthoracic sympathectomy: destroys the nerves that expand the tiny blood vessels in the face

Erectile dysfunction (impotence): inability to reach or maintain an erection of the penis sufficient for sex

Erectile tissue: three long cylinders in the penis with spongy inner portions. When blood flows in, the spongy portions swell up until the penis is erect

Erection: when erectile tissue in the penis becomes engorged with blood, making it swell and become hard

Estrogen: a hormone produced mainly by the ovaries in women

F **Feces:** also called stools. Waste matter that passes out of the body through the anus

Flatulence: a build-up of gas in the stomach or

bowels, which is released through the mouth as a burp or the anus as a fart

Foreskin: the fold of skin over the end of the penis (also known as the *prepuce*)

G

Galvanic stimulation: electrical stimulation

Genitals: the sexual organs that are visible between the legs

Gingivitis: gum disease – the gums are swollen and bleed easily

Gland: an organ or group of cells that produces a specific substance, e.g. the prostate gland produces part of the fluid that makes up semen

Gynaecomastia: overdevelopment of breasts in men

H

Halitophobia: delusion of halitosis – a psychological condition in which people believe that their breath smells, although it does not

Halitosis: bad breath

Hirsutism: excess hair growth

Hormone replacement therapy (HRT): the hormone estrogen to replace the falling levels at menopause. It can be in the form of tablets, patches, implants, vaginal creams or vaginal rings. In women who have not had a hysterectomy, progesterone must be taken as well for 10–14 days of the month, to prevent any increased risk of cancer of the womb

Hormones: chemicals produced by a gland in the body, and carried in the blood to other parts of the body where they have an effect. Examples are thyroxine produced by the thyroid gland, testosterone produced mainly by the testes in men, estrogen produced mainly by the ovaries in women, corticosteroids produced by the adrenal glands

Human papillomavirus (HPV): the virus that causes genital warts in humans

I

Impotence (erectile dysfunction): inability to reach or maintain an erection of the penis sufficient for sex

Incontinence of faeces: inability to control the passage of feces

Incontinence of urine: inability to control the passage of urine

Intertrigo: a red 'sweat rash' under the breasts

Inverted nipples: are tucked into the breast, instead of being flat or sticking out

Iontophoresis: use of an electric current to allow a drug to pass through the skin and reach a deep site

Irritable bladder: the muscle in the bladder starts to contract when it should be stretching to hold more urine

L

Leakage: slight incontinence of urine or feces

Libido: sexual desire

Ligation: 'tying off'. In surgery for varicose veins, the vein is tied off above the varicose section and the part of the vein below the tie is removed

M

Mastopexy: surgery to tighten up drooping breasts

Menopause: the time of the last period, usually between ages 45 and 55 – sometimes called the 'change of life'

Molluscum contagiosum: small lumps on the skin, each with a tiny dimple in the centre, caused by a virus, and transmitted by close body contact (usually sexual)

Morning-after pill: the old name for emergency contraception, which prevents pregnancy after sex has occurred. It can be taken up to 72 hours after intercourse

Muscle pump: the contractions of the leg muscles during walking force blood along the veins and back towards the heart

Myokymia: blepharospasm – uncontrollable twitching of the muscles around the eyes

N

Nabothian follicles: small glands, like pimples, on the cervix.

Non-cyclical breast pain: breast pain that has no monthly pattern

NSU: non-specific urethritis, an inflammation of the urethra. Symptoms are discharge and discomfort on passing urine. It is often caused by *Chlamydia* bacteria

P

Pelvic floor muscles: hold the bowel, uterus and bladder in place and help the bladder neck to keep the bladder closed

Peyronie's disease: the penis becomes crooked when it is erect

Phimosis: foreskin that is so tight that it cannot

be pulled back over the head of the penis

Polycystic ovary syndrome: cysts (small fluid-filled bags) develop on the ovary and hormone levels are disturbed, causing symptoms such as excess hair, acne and greasy hair, scanty or irregular periods or no periods at all

Postnasal drip: infected mucus that trickles down the back of the throat

Premature ejaculation: ejaculation occurring before the man or his partner wishes

Prepuce: the fold of skin over the end of the penis; also known as the foreskin

Proctalgia fugax: occasional, severe, cramp-like pain deep in the anal canal, lasting about half an hour

Prolapse: sagging of the walls of the vagina, or of the womb itself

Pudendal nerve: branches of this nerve go to the back passage and anus, and to the penis or clitoris

Receding hair: loss of hair at the sides of the forehead

Rectum: back passage – the last 12 cm (4 inches) of the large intestine, where the feces sit before they pass out of the body

Sclerotherapy: a solution is injected into a varicose vein. The solution causes irritation, inflammation and scarring, which permanently blocks the vein

Scrotum: the bag of skin that contains the testicles, which make the sperm

Seborrhoeic dermatitis: a skin disease – the skin is flaky and there are yellow crusts. The flaky areas are often on the scalp or face

Sexual disuse syndrome: difficulty in functioning sexually after a period of celibacy

Skin tag: a small lump found alongside an anal fissure (split in the anal skin)

Skin turnover: the skin renewal process. New skin cells form in the lower layers, are pushed to the surface, and then shed

Sleep apnea syndrome: a sleep disorder in which there are periods when breathing stops altogether for 10 seconds or more – the body's arousal system causes it to resume

Squeeze technique and stop–go technique: used to 'unlearn' premature ejaculation. Both techniques involve stimulating the penis almost to the point of ejaculation and then stopping

Stress incontinence: leaking of urine when you cough or laugh or bend over, or with exercise such as jumping or jogging

Stripping: a way of removing varicose veins. A tiny wire is used to pull the vein out through a small incision at the calf or ankle

Superficial veins: veins just under the skin

Telogen: the resting phase in hair development that occurs before the hair is shed

Testosterone: the main male hormone. Both men and women have testosterone, but men have more

Thrombosis: condition in which a blood clot develops

Urethra: the tube taking urine from the bladder to the outside

Urge incontinence: suddenly needing to pass urine desperately. People with urge incontinence may have to pass urine more than eight times a day, but may not pass much each time

Urologist: hospital doctor specializing in the urinary tract – some urologists are also experts in erection problems

Vaginismus: this is rare. It is when the muscles of the woman's vagina go into a spasm, and make her vagina seem too small for sex, when her partner tries to insert his penis. The woman cannot control the spasm

Valves: allow blood in the veins to flow in one direction only

Vulva: the fleshy area surrounding the openings of the vagina and the urethra

About the author

Dr Margaret Stearn qualified in medicine, with a
BA in Physiology and Psychology along the way,
from Oxford University and St George's Hospital
Medical School. She has had a varied medical
career and, until recently, worked in a busy
medical clinic. Here she developed a particular
interest in women's problems. Currently working in
a hospital diabetes clinic, Dr Stearn is also
Medical Commissioning Editor for *Medicine
International;* and contributed a regular medical
page to the magazine *Working Woman.*

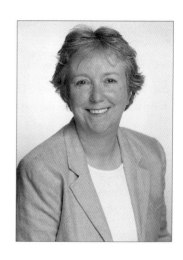

Ordering more copies

Embarrassing Medical Problems
For friends and family, old or young, male or female,
Embarrassing Medical Problems contains something for everyone.

US $14.95 each

You can order *Embarrassing Medical Problems* by phone, mail or E-mail.
Use the tear-out page opposite, or write to:
Hatherleigh Press
522 46th Avenue Suite 200, Long Island City, NY 11101
Phone: 800-528-2550, E-mail: info@hatherleighpress.com
http://www.hatherleighpress.com

Please make checks payable to Hatherleigh Press.
Prices are subject to change without notice.

Ordering more copies/suggestions for the second edition

Embarrassing Medical Problems

US$14.95 each

(please add $1.50 per copy for postage and packing)

Please send me ____copies of *Embarrassing Medical Problems*

I wish to pay by
☐ check   ☐ Amex   ☐ Mastercard   ☐ Visa   ☐ Discover

I enclose a check for US$ _____

I authorize you to debit my account with the amount of $ _____

Credit card number   __ __ __ __ __ __ __ __ __ __ __ __ __ __ __

Expiration date   __ __ __ __

Signature _____

Name   _____

Address   _____

_____

_____

Zipcode _____   Country _____

Telephone _____

Are there any problems you consider should be included in the next edition of *Embarrassing Medical Problems?* If so, please write them here:

....

Send this form and your check to: **Hatherleigh Press**

522 46th Avenue Suite 200, Long Island City, NY 11101

http://www.hatherleighpress.com

Please make checks payable to Hatherleigh Press.

Prices are subject to change without notice.

Please allow 21 days for delivery.